The
HEALTHY
KIDNEY
Handbook

The HEALTHY KIDNEY Handbook

A COMPREHENSIVE GUIDE TO Manage Hypertension, Control Stress, and Prevent Renal Failure, Kidney Disease, and More

C. NICOLE SWINER, MD

Text copyright © 2025 C. Nicole Swiner. Design and concept copyright © 2025 Ulysses Press and its licensors. All rights reserved. Any unauthorized duplication in whole or in part or dissemination of this edition by any means (including but not limited to photocopying, electronic devices, digital versions, and the internet) will be prosecuted to the fullest extent of the law.

Published by:
Ulysses Press
an imprint of The Stable Book Group
32 Court Street, Suite 2109
Brooklyn, NY 11201
www.ulyssespress.com

ISBN: 978-1-64604-767-3
Library of Congress Control Number: 2025930791

Printed in the United States
10 9 8 7 6 5 4 3 2 1

Acquisitions editor: Kierra Sondereker
Managing editor: Claire Chun
Editor: Renee Rutledge
Proofreader: Sherian Brown
Indexer: S4Carlisle Publishing Services
Front cover design: Amy King
Layout: Abbey Gregory
Artwork: cover © Chayon Sarker/Adobe Stock; page 9 © nmfotograf/Adobe Stock; page 12 © Designua/shutterstock.com.

NOTE TO READERS: This book has been written and published strictly for informational and educational purposes only. It is not intended to serve as medical advice or to be any form of medical treatment. You should always consult your physician before altering or changing any aspect of your medical treatment and/ or undertaking a diet regimen. Do not stop or change any prescription medications without the guidance and advice of your physician. Any use of the information in this book is made on the reader's good judgment after consulting with his or her physician and is the reader's sole responsibility. This book is not intended to diagnose or treat any medical condition and is not a substitute for a physician. This book is independently authored and published and no sponsorship or endorsement of this book by, and no affiliation with, any trademarked brands or other products mentioned within is claimed or suggested. All trademarks that appear in this book belong to their respective owners and are used here for informational purposes only.

Contents

Foreword.. ix

Introduction 1

Glossary 3

PART 1: THE FUNDAMENTALS OF KIDNEY HEALTH 5

Chapter 1: What Keeps the Kidneys Healthy?.......... 7
Anatomy of the Kidney 8
The Renin-Angiotensin System 11
What Can Keep Your Kidneys Healthy? 12

Chapter 2: Nutrition and Kidney Health................... 17
Vitamin A 17
Vitamin B9 (Folate) and B12 17
Vitamin C 18
Vitamin D.. 19
Vitamin E 21

Chapter 3: The Basics of Kidney Disease................ 23
What Is Renal Failure?... 23
Stages of Kidney Disease 24
Dialysis 28

Chapter 4: Drug Toxicity 33

Non-Steroidal Anti-Inflammatory Drugs (NSAIDs) 33

Antibiotics 34

Blood-Pressure Medications 36

Illegal Drugs 36

Tobacco and the Kidneys 38

Alcohol and the Kidneys 39

Chapter 5: Swelling 41

The IV Hydration Trend 42

PART 2: HEALTH CONDITIONS IMPACTING THE KIDNEYS 45

Chapter 6: Diabetes, or "the Sugars" 47

Prediabetes 47

Type 2 Diabetes and Kidney Disease 48

Weight-Loss Drugs and the Kidneys 50

Chapter 7: Hypertension 57

What Is Hypertension? 57

Natural Remedies for High Blood Pressure 58

Exercise and Blood Pressure 63

Sodium in Food 63

Massage and Its Effect on Blood Pressure 64

Hypertensive Crisis/Urgency/Emergency 65

The Classic Blood Pressure Meds 68

Chapter 8: Glomerular Diseases 73

Focal Segmental Glomerulosclerosis 74

Minimal Change Disease 76

Post-infectious Glomerulonephritis 77

Chapter 9: Autoimmune Diseases and the Kidney 79

Systemic Lupus Erythematosus 79

Rheumatoid Arthritis 82

Wegener's Granulomatosis 83

Goodpasture's Syndrome 84

Chapter 10: Adrenal Gland Issues 87

Adrenal Adenomas.. 87

Pheochromocytoma 89

Adrenal Fatigue.. 90

Adrenal Insufficiency 91

Chapter 11: Urinary Tract Infections 93

Pyelonephritis 95

Vesicoureteral Reflux 95

Kidney Stones.. 96

Chapter 12: COVID-19 and the Kidneys.......... 99

The Use of ACEIs and ARBs 102

Chapter 13: HIV and Kidney Disease 105

Chapter 14: Kidney Cysts and Polycystic Kidney Disease 109

Polycystic Kidney Disease.. 110

Chapter 15: Kidney Cancers.................... 113

Renal Cell Carcinoma.. 113

Angiomyolipoma of the Kidneys...................................... 114

PART 3: SPECIAL CIRCUMSTANCES.................. 117

Chapter 16: Kidney Transplants 119

A Personal Account.. 122

Chapter 17: Pregnancy and the Kidneys.......... 129

Dialysis During Pregnancy 131

Hypertension in Pregnancy... 132

Preeclampsia/Eclampsia.. 133

Q&A Section...137

Conclusion..141

Resources 143

References..145

Index 153

Acknowledgments...161

About the Author...163

Foreword

The Centers for Disease Control and Prevention defines a public health emergency as "an event that can cause harm to a person's health or to the health of a community." In our generation, this phrase undoubtedly raises heart-pounding memories of the COVID-19 pandemic that descended on our world with a thunderous roar in 2020. What if I told you that another public health emergency has been in our midst for years, long before the COVID pandemic? Rather than a thunderous roar, this public health emergency—the prevalence of kidney disease—has been stealthy and quiet, affecting over 37 million people in the US alone. What's even more alarming is that 9 out of 10 affected individuals have no idea they are a part of this number.[1]

No other organ in the body has a more crowded job description than the kidney. Admittedly, I may exhibit some bias as a kidney specialist, but I will always stand by that statement. Most people understand that the kidneys are responsible for filtering waste products and extra water from the bloodstream. In addition to that important role, the kidneys secrete hormones that play a major role in controlling blood pressure, balancing elec-

---

[1] National Institute of Diabetes and Digestive and Kidney Diseases, "Kidney Disease Statistics for the United States," May 2023, https://www.niddk.n h.gov/health -information/health-statistics/kidney-disease.

trolytes like sodium and potassium in the bloodstream, making sure red blood cells are being made in the bone marrow, converting vitamin D to a form the body can use to manage calcium and phosphorus levels in the blood and prevent weakening bones, balancing the pH of the bloodstream, and in children—supporting normal growth. How can a disease that affects an organ with so many functions in the body do so silently? With the exception of a few specific diseases, the symptoms of kidney disease are not obvious until you're in complete kidney failure, and often when it's too late to reverse the damage.

Kidney disease does not care if you barely finished high school or have a PhD. It does not care if you're a man or woman. Like so many chronic diseases, however, the burden of kidney disease disproportionately impacts communities of color—in particular Black and Hispanic communities. Kidney disease is overrepresented as well in rural areas.

Here's the good news: We have many tools in our arsenal to fight this silent threat, and knowledge is power. *The Healthy Kidney Handbook* provides the information we all need to understand these tools in a perfectly organized and easy-to-digest format.

I am by no means an accidental nephrologist. As a Black woman raised in the South, I come from a very large family that has been heavily impacted by kidney disease. It has been my personal passion to see tools like *The Healthy Kidney Handbook* empower our communities to fight back against this epidemic of kidney disease.

For more than 20 years, I have been proud to know Dr. Swiner as an amazing physician, mom, wife, author, media personality, champion for self-care, and friend. I will be recommending this latest work to everyone I know and care about.

—Keisha L. Gibson, MD

Keisha L. Gibson, MD, is clinical associate professor of medicine and pediatrics and chief of pediatric nephrology in the Division of Nephrology and Hypertension at the University of North Carolina at Chapel Hill.

***

Kidney.org mentions that kidney disease is a leading cause of death in the US. I work in Baltimore, Maryland, where complications from kidney disease fall within the top 10 causes of mortality in adults. As a family physician practicing in this environment, I daily treat patients with complications from diabetes, hypertension, and the like, and I'm always concerned about their long-term kidney health. In the US, Black adults are four times more likely to suffer from kidney failure than their White counterparts, and make up an estimated 30% of patients receiving dialysis.[2] Recognizing the vast health disparities in conditions leading to kidney disease, especially working in a city whose population is overwhelmingly comprised of historically marginalized individuals, I believe this book will help put ways into layman's terms for kidneys to be more protected for longer and prevent patients from having to deal with chronic kidney disease and, ultimately, failure.

---

2 Centers for Disease Control and Prevention, "Chronic Kidney Disease in the United States, 2021," accessed July 24, 2024, https://nccd.cdc.gcv/CKD/Documents/Chronic-Kidney-Disease-in-the-US-2021-h.pdf.

I've known Dr. Swiner for almost 15 years—first as my attending physician, then as my primary care provider, then soon after as a lifelong friend and mentor. I plan to use this as a guide for my patients to understand more about their health and how to live longer, healthier lives.

—Kristin Powell Reavis, MD

Kristin Powell Reavis, MD, is a family medicine obstetric clinician and a clinical assistant professor in the Department of Family and Community Medicine at University of Maryland School of Medicine (UMSOM). She is also a director of the Family Medicine Residency program, the assistant dean for student diversity and inclusion, and a director of maternal child health at UMSOM.

Introduction

My journey to becoming a board-certified family physician included the study of many topics in various disciplines, including pediatrics, nephrology, urology and gastrointestinal medicine, to name a few. One organ that encompasses all of those areas that I've always loved (and even considered focusing solely on in practice) is the kidney. I was always impressed at the way it works and fascinated by the many different processes that can go wrong both inside and outside of the organ. Understanding this organ really does enlighten you on almost any disease process, from diabetes to heart failure to infections.

But I'm not just interested in how kidneys are afflicted with illness. I'm even more interested in what keeps many of us from maintaining our kidney health. Why is it so hard to control our salt intake, drink enough water, and refrain from smoking or using substances that harm us? We'll delve a little into those topics here, as well.

The Centers for Disease Control (CDC) indicates that chronic kidney disease (CKD) affects more than 1 in 7 US adults–about 35.5 million people, or 14% of Americans as of 2023. CKD is more common in non-Hispanic Black adults (20%) than in non-Hispanic Asian or Hispanic adults (both at 14%) or non-Hispanic White adults (12%).[3] One of my goals with this book is to help dispel the myths that cause such discrepancies between racial groups and decrease the gap in terms of access to knowledge and to better preventive health, in general, and specifically, for kidney-related health conditions.

Why is it that this and many other health conditions tend to affect populations of color more than White populations? Is it genetic, environmental, or social? Does it involve access to affordable and equitable health care, or discrimination and a lack of diversity and inclusion within the industry? It is likely a combination of all the above. As the medical field works harder to increase inclusion on the medical research side of things and humanity recognizes the disheartening reality of racism and how it has affected the health and health care of disenfranchised communities, we are all recognizing what needs to happen to improve the lives of all patients, regardless of background. This also applies to kidney disease.

Unfortunately, over five hundred thousand patients nationwide still require dialysis each year.[4] Dialysis for one patient usually occurs multiple times a week, usually at a dialysis center, for at least 15 to 20 years. If they start in their twenties, this can equate to almost one hundred thousand dollars in medical expenses. What we do *before* they are afflicted and to prevent high blood pressure, diabetes, or cancers helps to bring those numbers down. This includes

---

3 Centers for Disease Control and Prevention, "Chronic Kidney Disease in the United States, 2023."

4 Muhammad F. Hashmi, Onecia Benjamin, and Sarah L. Lappin, *End-Stage Renal Disease* (Treasure Island: StatPearls Publishing, 2023), https://www.ncbi.nlm.nih.gov /books/NBK499861.

counseling on good nutrition, ridding communities of food deserts, teaching low-sodium food options at younger ages, decreasing unhealthy fast food intake, improving access to consistent exercise, and doing better to combat nicotine and alcohol overuse in the United States.

Glossary

Here are some words and/or phrases to become familiar with before reading:

Adrenal glands. These sit atop each organ and produce hormones that regulate key bodily functions, like metabolism and reproduction.

Diabetes. There are two or more recognizable types of diabetes. In this book, I'm largely referring to type 2.

Hypertensive urgency. A clinical scenario where blood pressure is significantly elevated (e.g., 220/125 mmHg) but the patient exhibits minimal or no symptoms and shows no signs of acute organ damage.

Hypertensive emergency. Severely high blood pressure accompanied by evidence of progressive damage to organs or bodily systems.

Kidney. Often interchangeable with "renal." At times, I may refer to the kidney as one or two separate organs.

Renin-angiotensin system. One of the most important systems of kidney function, which handles the creation and balance of important electrolytes and hormones.

Introduction

Renal failure. Related to the fifth stage of chronic kidney disease or end-stage renal disease.

Renal insufficiency. Poor function of the kidney.

Sugar/the Sugars. When I say "sugar," I generally mean glucose. "The Sugars" is a colloquialism sometimes used to describe type 2 diabetes.

The explanations and opinions contained herein are mine, unless I reference an actual study, textbook, or organization. This book is in no way one to be used for self-diagnosing or self-management. It is for understanding. Please take your specific concerns to your medical professional to discuss further.

Ultimately, I want this book to help you get to a healthier state, stay healthy, prevent disease, and better understand the conditions that may be plaguing you or your loved ones. Thank you for choosing this resource. Let's get started!

PART 1

THE FUNDAMENTALS OF KIDNEY HEALTH

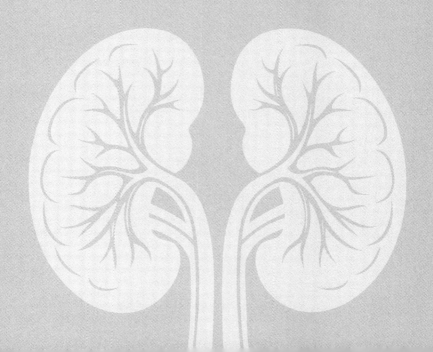

CHAPTER 1

What Keeps the Kidneys Healthy?

"In the Old Testament most frequently the kidneys are associated with the most inner stirrings of emotional life. But they are also viewed as the seat of the secret thoughts of the human; they are used as an omen metaphor, as a metaphor for moral discernment, for reflection and inspiration."[5]

—Giovanni Maio

What came first...the organ or the bean?

It was the organ, clearly.

Could there have been theories that the kidneys rivaled the heart as the most important organ system in the human body? It certainly seems like it. As it turns out, the kidneys are extremely important.

I am a Southern girl, so I always think of kidney beans when I think of the organ! Well, as important as the kidney bean is to so many of our recipes, so are the organs to the total function of the human (and animal, for that matter) body. Many stories and myths are written about these two bean-shaped organs that lie near our backs, under the end of the rib cage. If you google it, you'll find

---

5 Giovanni Maio, "The Metaphorical and Mythical Use of the Kidney in Antiquity," *American Journal of Nephrology* 19, no. 2 (January 1, 1999): 101–6, https://doi.org/10.1159/000013434.

references to kidneys spanning from the Old Testament to Michaelangelo. Most of us have two kidneys, but some of us may have one *U*-shaped or uni-kidney. (And, yes, people can live successfully with just one functioning kidney.) Some may even have lost or donated a kidney and now rely on one really strong kidney. However many you have, the kidney's primary job is to be the filtration system of the body. What we eat, drink, or put into our bodies is filtered through the kidneys into the urine. And, that's an incredibly important function to be responsible for.

As adults, we each produce urine at a rate of about 20 to 30 milliliters per hour (ml/hr), equaling about 800 to 1200 ml per day.[6] Any more or less than that may depend on one's hydration status, which is why adequate water intake is so important.

Anatomy of the Kidney

As mentioned, most people have two kidneys in the body, and they are located in the abdominal cavity near the back. They almost hug the two largest blood vessels that run through the body: the aorta and the inferior vena cava (IVC). They are connected to the back by connective tissue that holds them in place, so they don't float around, and each has a ureter that connects them to the bladder. Each kidney has a renal artery that supplies blood to the kidney from the heart and a vein that returns the blood and products to the heart.

---

6 Nancy C. Tkacs, Linda H. Herrmann, and Blair Thielemier, *Advanced Physiology and Pathophysiology: Essentials for Clinical Practice* (New York: Springer Publishing, 2020).

Adrenal Glands

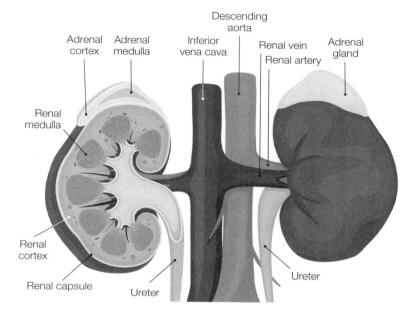

There is a small gland, called the adrenal gland, that sits atop each organ. These "top hats" of your kidneys produce hormones, like cortisol, aldosterone, and the "sex hormones" estrogen and androgen. Part of the endocrine system, the hormones produced by the adrenal glands regulate key bodily functions, like metabolism and reproduction. These hormones are created in the outer adrenal cortex and inner adrenal medulla layers of each adrenal gland, which is encapsulated by a protective covering.

Adrenaline-Related Hormones

- Epinephrine, or adrenaline, is released during acute stress, such as sudden shock or fear. It triggers a variety of physiological changes, including increased heart rate, blood pressure, and blood sugar levels.

- Similarly, norepinephrine, or noradrenaline, tightens blood vessels, which can have the same effects.[7]

Glucocorticoids and Sex Hormones

- Aldosterone helps the kidneys regulate the body's salt and fluid balance by controlling the amount of sodium, potassium, and water in the blood and tissues.

- Cortisol plays a crucial role in the body's metabolism. It helps the body manage and utilize carbohydrates, proteins, and fats. It also triggers changes in metabolism to assist the body in managing stress, and it can suppress the immune system.

- Androgens are male sex hormones produced by the adrenal glands in both men and women, though in different amounts. These hormones are responsible for the growth, development, and functioning of the reproductive organs. Androgens also control the development of male physical characteristics, such as a deep voice, body and facial hair growth (hirsutism), and body shape. Importantly, androgens are necessary for the production of estrogen. Estrogen is a female sex hormone that regulates female reproduction and sexual development, including the growth of breasts and other female physical traits.

Once you understand the parts of the kidney, it's much easier to understand its function and how diseases affect it.

---

7 "Adrenal Gland Hormones," Canadian Cancer Society, accessed July 24, 2024, https://cancer.ca/en/cancer-information/cancer-types/adrenal-gland/what-is-adrenal-gland-cancer/adrenal-gland-hormones.

The Renin-Angiotensin System

Along with the anatomy of the kidneys, the renin-angiotensin system, which handles the creation and balance of important electrolytes and hormones, is, by far, one of the most important cycles to understand as far as the function of the kidneys is concerned. This fairly complicated chart that you see here explains how the different hormones of the kidney interact and counteract one another, when it comes to how blood pressure, fluids, and electrolytes are all balanced.[8]

This chart also shows where the major medications that treat blood pressure (i.e., the ACE [angiotensin-converting enzyme]-inhibitors and ARBs [angiotensin receptor blockers]), interplay with the system and help block the buildup of the negative chemicals that cause elevated pressures. We'll talk more about the specific medicines in Chapter 9. You should also know that sodium chloride, or salt, is noted as NaCl on the periodic table (remember that from high school chemistry?]. Na alone is sodium. The renin-angiotensin system chart shows how important it is to the renin-angiotensin cycle, which is why we have to watch our sodium and salty food intake to help prevent renal issues. The maximum amount of daily sodium intake should match the year. So, in general, try to limit daily intake to about 2025-ish milligrams (mg) per day. If you look it up, it's actually about 2300 mg per day for most

---

8 Amandeep Goyal, Austin S. Cusick, and Blair Thielemier, *ACE Inhibitors* (Treasure Island: StatPearls Publishing, 2023), https://www.ncbi.nlm.nih.gov/books/NBK430896/figure/article-17070.image.f1.

adults. For children or those with certain health conditions, the amount is lower.[9]

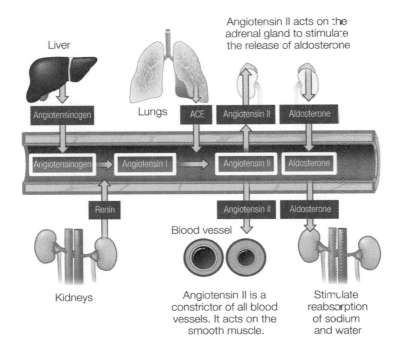

What Can Keep Your Kidneys Healthy?

This book will focus on many of the conditions, illnesses, and health problems that affect the kidneys, but what's most important is figuring out what keeps your kidneys most healthy. Keeping your kidneys healthy is essential for overall well-being, as they play a crucial role in filtering

---

[9] American Heart Association Staff, "How Much Sodium Should I Eat Per Day?" Heart.org, last modified January 5, 2024, https://www.heart.org/en/healthy-living/healthy-eating/eat-smart/sodium/how-much-sodium-should-i-eat-per-day.

waste and excess fluids from the body, maintaining electrolyte balance, and regulating blood pressure.

By making the healthy lifestyle choices outlined below, you can reduce your risk of kidney disease and promote better overall health.

- **Focus on adequate hydration.** To support kidney health, it's important to stay well-hydrated by drinking enough water throughout the day, as dehydration can strain kidney function. We'll touch more on hydration later, but in general, focus on at least 48 to 64 ounces of water a day to keep the body hydrated and flushed.

- **Limit sodium and salty foods.** Eating a balanced diet rich in fruits, vegetables, and whole grains, while limiting salt and processed foods, can help prevent kidney damage.

- **Avoid and/or quit tobacco intake and limit alcohol use.** Both alcohol and tobacco negatively impact the kidney's ability to filter, hastening renal failure.

- **Avoid and/or quit toxic substances.** The overuse of over-the-counter medications, prescription medications, and illegal drugs will also impact renal function.

- **Control your blood pressure.** Smoking tobacco and inhaling nicotine can negatively impact the effectiveness of medications used to manage high blood pressure, which is a leading cause of kidney disease.

- **Exercise regularly.** The kidneys definitely love regular exercise. What is regular exercise for an average adult? The Department of Health and Human Services recommends getting at least 150 minutes of moderate aerobic activity a week.[10] You can break that up into five days a week for 30 minutes of cardiovascular exercise (this usually translates to sweat on your brow and increased heart rate and respiratory rate). Or, three days a week for 50 minutes. Or, even every day of the week for about 20 minutes...whatever works for your schedule.

- **Decrease abnormal protein levels with your intake** (e.g., from meat, protein shakes, supplements).

- **Keep your blood sugar (glucose) normal.**

- **Control your weight and prevent or treat obesity.** With increased weight, all of the organs of our body, including the kidneys, have to carry the weight and work against more pressure. This can cause damage, which is why we focus on BMI, or body mass index, often, in medicine. If your BMI is > 35–40%, you should focus on how to get down to a healthier weight with lifestyle changes and physical activity.

- **Finally, check your renal function routinely,** particularly if you're at high risk for kidney disease.

In general, doing all of the things you know you should do–eating a balanced diet full of fruits and vegetables, avoiding too much sodium intake, drinking more water than caffeinated or sugary beverages, and staying away

---

10 U.S. Department of Health and Human Services, *Physical Activity Guidelines for Americans, 2nd Edition* (Washington, DC: U.S. Department of Health and Human Services, 2018), https://health.gov/sites/default/files/2019-09/Physical_Activity _Guidelines_2nd_edition.pdf.

from toxic and harmful items—keeps your kidneys healthier for a longer time.

If you check your blood urea nitrogen (BUN) and creatinine (we'll discuss these blood levels more in subsequent chapters) regularly, you can see if and when there is a "bump" or elevation that happens. If it's a small rise but only a couple of tenths of a point, generally speaking, the damage can be reversed before it becomes a chronic, irreversible issue.

The key is to prevent as many of the preventable diseases that can lead to kidney disease as possible by staying healthy. We'll discuss many of those diseases in this book. There are some you can't control, meaning they are related to genetic predisposition and family history, so do your best to protect your health.

CHAPTER 2

Nutrition and Kidney Health

Many vitamin deficiencies or anemias are actually a consequence of kidney disease. However, when it comes to preventing kidney problems, it's important to be mindful of certain vitamins that, when taken in excess, can potentially harm kidney function.

Vitamin A

One key vitamin to watch is vitamin A. High doses of this fat-soluble vitamin can accumulate in the body and lead to toxicity, which may cause kidney damage over time.

Vitamin B9 (Folate) and B12

These are essential for overall health, particularly for red blood cell production and DNA synthesis, but their effects on kidney health can vary depending on individual circumstances. Vitamin B9 plays a role in regulating homocysteine levels in the blood, an amino acid that, when elevated, can contribute to kidney damage and cardiovascular disease. For individuals with pre-existing kidney conditions, low levels of folate may exacerbate these risks. Vitamin B12, on the other hand, is involved in nerve function and the production of red blood cells. While deficiency in B12 can lead to anemia and neurological issues, excessive intake, particularly in the form of high-dose supplements, could potentially worsen kidney function in individuals with chronic kidney disease (CKD). This is because the body may have difficulty excreting the excess vitamin, which could lead to toxicity in some cases.

In general, when managed properly through diet or supplementation, both vitamins B9 and B12 are important for kidney health, but it's crucial to avoid excessive doses, especially in individuals already at risk for kidney problems. Always consult a healthcare provider before making significant changes to vitamin intake.[11]

Vitamin C

Vitamin C is another one to be cautious with. While it's beneficial in moderate amounts, very high doses can cause kidney stones in susceptible individuals. To safeguard kidney health, it's best to avoid taking large doses of these vitamins unless specifically recommended by a healthcare provider, and to focus on obtaining nutrients from a balanced diet.

---

[11] Irene Capelli et al., "Folic Acid and Vitamin B12 Administration in CKD, Why Not?" *Nutrients* 11, no. 2 (February 2019): 383, 10.3390/nu11020383. PMID: 30781775; PMCID: PMC6413093.

Vitamin D

Vitamin D2 and D3 have become increasingly important and trendy topics, especially since the height of the COVID-19 pandemic, when we were stuck at home and not getting outside as much. With the decrease in sun exposure came lower vitamin D levels. (A normal amount of vitamin D, when checked in the bloodstream, is generally above 30 ng/dL.) Vitamin D deficiency is related to symptoms like chronic fatigue, low mood, low immune systems, and low bone density, or osteoporosis.

The kidney is important to the production of vitamin D, in tandem with our skin (our largest organ) and the liver. The inactive form of vitamin D, called 1,25-dihydroxyvitamin D (calcitriol), is created first in the skin from a molecule related to cholesterol, then transferred to the liver and finally to the kidney as calcitriol to help balance levels of phosphorus and calcium. The skin is activated initially by the ultraviolet rays from the sun.

People with melanin have trouble maintaining a normal level of vitamin D, often due to decreased absorption of ultraviolet rays from the skin, because the melanin is protective in blocking it. So, if the diet is lacking in intake of vitamin D and the skin is not able to absorb the needed energy it needs from being outside, it is always challenging to keep vitamin D levels elevated.

Vitamin D should be carefully monitored, especially in individuals with existing kidney disease, as excessive levels can result in calcium buildup in the kidneys, leading to kidney stones or impaired kidney function.

Treatment of Vitamin D Deficiency

As with any vitamin deficiency, dietary intake is always the most efficient and lasting treatment.

Foods that can increase vitamin D include:[12]

- Fatty fish
- Herring and sardines
- Cod liver oil
- Canned tuna
- Egg yolks
- Mushrooms
- Cow and soy milk
- Orange juice
- Cereal and oatmeal

We should all aim to get 800 IU (international units) of vitamin D daily, either in food and/or supplements. In practice, once a patient is diagnosed with a low vitamin D level (insufficiency, meaning levels < 21–29, or deficiency, meaning < 20), prescription vitamin D is usually initiated. An oral capsule of vitamin D3 (better absorbed orally than D2) of either 1000, 2000, 5000, or sometimes 50,000 IU is prescribed, depending on how low the level is. Vitamin D3 capsules and liquid are available over the counter and online, and generally a daily intake of 2000–5000 IU is enough to take. The 50,000 IU capsule is only available by

---

12 The Nutrition Source, "Vitamin D," March 2023, https://nutritionsource.hsph.harvard.edu/vitamin-d.

prescription and is usually taken once a week for a total of eight weeks and rechecked in three months. It takes that long to see a difference, for the most part.

Recently, IM (intramuscular) and IV (intravenous) applications have become viable options, because most things, if not through food absorbed in the gut, are best absorbed through the muscle or the veins. Have you ever noticed your oral multivitamins in the toilet after you've used the bathroom? That's because most vitamins taken orally, and even some medications, slide right through the stomach to the intestines and out in our waste. If given as an injection, or shot, or given through an IV treatment, it goes straight to where it's needed most–the soft tissues, the bloodstream, and to the organs. IM and IV doses can also be administered less frequently, meaning they likely last longer in the system, and can be more convenient for patients.

Vitamin E

Vitamin E, although an antioxidant, can also be problematic in high doses, potentially increasing the risk of bleeding and affecting kidney health.

Nutrition and Kidney Health

CHAPTER 3

The Basics of Kidney Disease

What Is Renal Failure?

The terms "renal failure" and "renal insufficiency" are often used interchangeably, which can be confusing for many people. However, when "renal insufficiency" is used, this generally means poor function of the kidney, whereas, renal failure is usually related to the fifth stage of CKD, or end-stage renal disease (ESRD).[13] (See CKD Stages on page 27.)

During any kind of kidney insult or injury, there is the potential for decreased function of the kidney–whether short term or long term. This decreased function can be associated with an elevated creatinine (Cr) level, which you can see in your labs, due to damage of the organ's tubules and glomeruli because of a variety of causes. You can also see an increase in two other numbers, called BUN, or blood urea nitrogen, and glomerular filtration rate (GFR), or the rate at which toxins are filtered through the kidneys.

---

[13] "Creatinine Blood Test," MountSinai.org, last modified August 20, 2023, https://www.mountsinai.org/health-library/tests/creatinine-blood-test.

But creatinine seems to be used more widely by medical practitioners as an indicator number. Acute renal failure (ARF) is when the damage is reversible and the function returns to baseline, or at least an improved level close to the patient's baseline. Chronic renal failure (CRF) is when the damage is persistent or irreversible and the creatinine level does not recover, and even worsens over time.

Depending on the lab and its ranges, a normal creatinine level is measured in the blood as between 0.7 and 1.3 mg/dL for adult men and 0.6 and 1.1 mg/dL for adult women. When levels rise by about 0.2 mg/dL for one reason or another and stays that way, we call it renal insufficiency and consider this abnormal. The investigation should begin to assess reasons why the number changed. We'll discuss the most common reasons and causes for renal failure in the following chapters.

Acute renal injury is treated depending on the issue that caused it, such as an infection, toxic drug effect, or dehydration. When treated, in time, hopefully normal function can be restored. However, if there is too much time between the injury and finding and treating the initial problem or the patient takes too long to seek treatment, the normal function of the organs may not be restored. The patient's baseline creatinine may now always be at a higher level and can worsen over time.

Stages of Kidney Disease

Acute kidney injury (or damage or failure) can be broken down in the following categories:

- **Prerenal**—when the insult has occurred outside of the kidney, affecting its function;
- **(Intra)Renal**—when the insult has occurred on the inside of the kidney (e.g., its tubules, receptors, etc.)
- **Postrenal**—when the insult has occurred on the outside of the kidney, affecting its output and function to the outside of the body.

When you think "prerenal," think of things that can prevent adequate blood flow and supply to the kidneys, such as problems with blood pressure, bleeding, burns, dehydration, infections, and drugs and medications. Renal causes of ARF should bring to mind intrinsic things, like blood clots (thrombosis), health conditions like lupus or glomerulonephritis (discussed more in subsequent chapters), alcohol damage, COVID-19, and blood disorders. Postrenal causes, occurring outside of the kidney, include stones, cancers, blood clots in the urinary tract, and anything that obstructs the flow of urine out of the kidneys or urinary tract.[14]

Symptoms of acute renal failure include difficulty with urination (either too much, known as urinary frequency or polyuria–or too little, known as urinary retention), painful urination (called dysuria), blood in the urine (hematuria), leg swelling or swelling of the face or body, weakness, confusion, and in severe cases, coma.

Once the creatinine and BUN levels are checked in the blood and a urine dip or urinalysis is assessed,

---

14 Shaziya Allarakha, "What Are the 3 Types of Acute Renal Failure? Symptoms, Treatment," MedicineNet.com, last updated January 5, 2022, https://www.medicinenet.com/what_are_the_3_types_of_acute_renal_failure/article.htm.

the cause of the failure can be identified. Or, at least a list of causes can be created in a differential, which is what medical professionals call their list of possible diagnoses. And, once the cause is identified, treatment can hopefully begin to reverse the damage, or preserve as much remaining function as is possible. What also can be helpful is calculating the BUN to creatinine ratio, because the number can tell you if the cause is prerenal, renal, or postrenal.

BUN TO CREATININE RATIO

RATIO	DESCRIPTION
> 20 to 1	Prerenal cause
12 – 20 to 1	Normal or postrenal cause
< 12 to 1	Intrarenal cause

Depending on the cause, treatment will follow, including IV fluids, withdrawing or discontinuing medications, starting different medications, using antibiotics, or removing an obstruction. In severe, emergent cases, short-term dialysis may need to occur. Hopefully, in a matter of hours or days, the creatinine will decrease and return to its baseline level. In chronic cases, where the damage to the kidneys has been prolonged or irreversible, chronic kidney disease can occur. Elevated creatinine levels are used to determine the severity, as well as the GFR.

CKD STAGES

Stage	DESCRIPTION	GFR
1	Normal or High	> 90 mL/min
2	Mild CKD	60–89 mL/min
3A	Moderate CKD	45–59 mL/min
3B	Moderate CKD	30–44 mL/min
4	Severe CKD	15–29 mL/min
5	End Stage CKD	<15 mL/min

It generally takes between two and five years for one stage to progress to the next stage, which means there's time to try to delay or even stop the worsening of the function, with the help of your doctors.

Stage 1 or 2 disease may or may not have any symptoms at all, which is why it's important to get your labs checked regularly, especially if you're at high risk. Treatment usually includes changing your habits, like diet and exercise, and removing any unnecessary toxins (drugs, alcohol, increased sodium, tobacco) from your intake to preserve kidney function. Regulating your blood pressure and blood sugar, if they are elevated, is often stressed.[15]

Stage 3 disease can be divided into 3a and 3b, depending on the GFR rate. At this point, elevated blood pressure and anemia are common symptoms. Anemia can be related to the decreased production of iron, a loss of blood iron, or the decreased production of red blood cells, also called "erythropoiesis." A medicine called Epo, which stimulates

---

15 Gian Maria Ladarola et al., "Is the Cost of the New Home Dialysis Techniques Still Advantageous Compared to In-Center Hemodialysis? An Italian Single Center Analysis and Comparison with Experiences from Western Countries," *Frontiers in Medicine* 11 (March 11, 2024), https://doi.org/10.3389/fmed.2024.1345506.

the glycoprotein cytokine erythropoietin, is prescribed sometimes to increase the production of blood cells or iron. It can be prescribed either orally or through IV administration. If a patient isn't already seeing a kidney specialist, called a nephrologist, along with your primary care team, this is the time to start.

Stage 4 is the level of damage right before full-on failure. Along with symptoms mentioned in Stage 3, bone disease can also occur.

Stage 5 is end-stage renal failure, and symptoms can include loss of appetite, trouble sleeping, muscle pain, and itching. Once at this stage, dialysis or transplant are the options to consider for survival. The key in all stages is to prevent worsening and movement into the next stage with the right management.

Dialysis

Once you've hit the end stage of renal disease and your kidneys are no longer producing or releasing urine normally, hemodialysis or dialysis becomes an option, and often a necessary, life-saving, and expensive one at that. It replaces the action of the kidneys and bladder for urine and toxin removal from the body. Some patients at this point may produce a small amount of urine and can eliminate it through the bladder, but most lose this action altogether.

The planning stages start way before reaching stage 5, including talks of and oftentimes moving forward with vein mapping and incising arteriovenous (AV) fistulas onto the arms for easier access to the bloodstream.

These access points, which are large, raised blood vessel channels on the arms of many dialysis patients, are usually surgically placed at least six months before the first dialysis treatment begins.

If dialysis is needed emergently and acutely in the hospital, there's no time to place an AV fistula, so a large hemodialysis machine is used with IVs and tubes in the arms to filter the blood out of the body, remove toxins, and return the blood without toxins back to the body. If you are a chronic dialysis patient, you either go to a dialysis center three or so days a week and sit to have this done through your fistula for an average of four hours.

Some patients are able to choose to do this at home, usually through the abdomen, through a process called "peritoneal dialysis." So, instead of having the AV fistulas on the arms, they create similar access through the abdomen. The patient plugs into their equipment at home and has the process completed there instead of a clinic.

Dialysis can sometimes be a painful, cold process. The process of the filtration of blood is generally painless, but the side effects can include nausea, vomiting, muscle cramping, and occasionally seizures. Patients will continue to need very close follow-up with their renal specialists, primary care provider, and dialysis center (if they attend in-person) providers. In few instances, patients can recover from chronic dialysis and can have use of their own kidney function again depending on significant treatment.

Of note, the typical in-clinic dialysis session costs between $250 and $350, with most patients requiring three sessions per week. In contrast, home-based peritoneal dialysis, while slightly less expensive, still carries an estimated annual cost of $53,000 to $65,000.[16]

Hemodialysis vs. Peritoneal Dialysis

Hemodialysis involves using an external machine to filter waste and excess fluid from the blood. The blood is drawn from the body, filtered through a dialyzer (artificial kidney), and then returned to the body.[17]

Pros:

- **Efficient Filtration:** Hemodialysis can remove larger amounts of waste and fluid in a shorter amount of time.

- **Regular Monitoring:** Dialysis centers are staffed with healthcare professionals who monitor the process, reducing the risk of complications during treatment.

- **Less Daily Maintenance:** Treatments are typically done three times a week, allowing for days without dialysis.

- **Best for Acute Cases:** Hemodialysis is often used for patients with acute kidney failure or those who need immediate treatment.

Cons:

- **Time and Schedule:** Treatment usually takes three to five hours per session and is often needed three times

---

16 Cleveland Clinic, "Granulomatosis with Polyangiitis (GPA, Formerly Called Wegener's)," last updated July 16, 2019, https://my.clevelandclinic.org/health/diseases/4757 -granulomatosis-with-polyangiitis-gpa-formerly-called-wegeners.

17 Cleveland Clinic, "Dialysis," last updated August 18, 2021, https://my.clevelandclinic .org/health/treatments/14618-dialysis.

per week. This can interfere with work, school, and personal activities.

- **Access Issues:** A permanent access point, like an arteriovenous (AV) fistula, graft, or central venous catheter, is needed for blood to be removed and returned, which can increase the risk of infections and clotting.

- **Potential for Low Blood Pressure:** Hemodialysis can cause rapid shifts in fluid balance, potentially leading to hypotension (low blood pressure), dizziness, or fainting.

- **Diet and Fluid Restrictions:** Patients on hemodialysis must adhere to strict diet and fluid intake restrictions to avoid complications.

Peritoneal dialysis uses the lining of the abdomen (the peritoneum) as a natural filter. A dialysis solution is introduced into the peritoneal cavity, where it absorbs waste and excess fluids, and is then drained.[18]

Pros:

- **More Independence:** Peritoneal dialysis can often be done at home, and many patients can perform the procedure themselves. There's also the option for automated peritoneal dialysis (APD) during sleep.

- **Gentler on the Body:** The process is continuous and tends to be more gentle than hemodialysis. It is less likely to cause sudden changes in blood pressure.

- **No Need for Blood Access:** Since the treatment uses the peritoneum as a filter, there is no need for a

---

18 Cleveland Clinic, "Dialysis."

The Basics of Kidney Disease

permanent vascular access point, lowering the risk of infection or clotting.

- **Flexible Scheduling:** Patients can adjust the timing of their dialysis, allowing for more flexibility compared to the rigid schedule of hemodialysis.

Cons:

- **Potential for Infection:** The risk of infection (peritonitis) is a major concern, especially if proper hygiene is not maintained during the exchange process.

- **Space Requirements:** You need a clean, dry space to store dialysis supplies, and the process may require a dedicated area in the home.

- **Longer Treatment Duration:** Each dialysis exchange typically takes around thirty minutes, but because it's done more frequently (often every day), it can be time-consuming.

- **Fluid Overload Risk:** As there is a smaller amount of dialysis solution in use compared to hemodialysis, some people may not achieve the same level of fluid and waste removal, potentially leading to fluid overload.

- **Not Suitable for Everyone:** People with severe abdominal conditions or previous abdominal surgeries may not be candidates for peritoneal dialysis, as the peritoneum may not function as effectively.

CHAPTER 4

Drug Toxicity

We use medications for a great many reasons, and amazing advancements in medicine have been made over the decades. However, we have to recognize the downside of medications—the adverse side effects. Over-the-counter medicines can be misused or overused, or sometimes, the body can react negatively to prescribed medication. All in all, we have to be careful and closely monitor the things we put in our bodies for those adverse effects, known and silent, that can happen over time to the kidneys.

Non-Steroidal Anti-Inflammatory Drugs (NSAIDs)

Outside of acetaminophen (Tylenol), NSAIDs like ibuprofen (Advil, Motrin), naproxen (Aleve, Naprosyn), and aspirin are the most commonly known and used medications used for pain, inflammation, and fever. Some patients already know they are allergic to these types of medicines, but if taken in higher dosages than recommended, these medicines can cause interstitial nephritis (inflammation and damage of the tubules) and pyelonephritis (infection). Symptoms of adverse reactions of the kidneys to these drugs can include blood in the urine and a rise in creatinine levels, as seen in blood work. For ibuprofen, the maximum dose for adults that should be taken is 800 mg every three hours, and, for naproxen, the maximum dose is 660 mg in a day. Too much NSAID intake can irritate the stomach and GI tract and cause bleeding and ulceration, as well.

Don't forget our favorite little over-the-counter packets for pain or headaches, like Excedrin, Goody's powders, BC powders, and Stanback powders, all of which include aspirin, too. Don't overuse them without talking to your doctors about it.

Antibiotics

Medicines used to treat infection unfortunately can also cause harm. Notably, the floroquinolones, like levafloxacin or ciprofloxacin, have to be monitored for those with known kidney disease. Even if taken as prescribed, there is a risk for acute renal failure. That is one among many of the reasons that prescribers should be and generally are concerned about prescribing too many antibiotics or prescribing them for unnecessary situations.

The cephalosporin class of antibiotics is widely used and includes examples like cefuroxime (Ceftin), ceftriaxone (Rocephin) and cephalexin (Keflex), prescribed for gram-positive bacterial infections, from streptococcal pharyngitis (strep throat), to UTIs, to skin infections (cellulitis). These antibiotics are used daily by patients. The danger to the kidneys comes with the potential damage that can be done to the tubules. This effect seems to be dose-dependent, meaning the higher the dose, the higher the risk of damage.

The aminoglycoside class of antibiotics that includes tobramycin and gentamycin, more commonly used via IV and in the hospital, are very toxic to the kidneys. So is vancomycin, which is similar to the aminoglycosides but treats different bacteria. These antibiotics are used for serious and severe bacterial infections from gram-negative and gram-positive bacteria, and they can damage the kidney by causing damage to its small tubules, potentially leading to chronic kidney disease.

All in all, antibiotics, in general, should be used judiciously and with caution. They are wonderful drugs that treat bacterial infections and save lives, but the risk of organ damage and allergic reactions is a real thing, and doctors consider this every day when treating their patients. Side note: next time you have a "cold," "sinus infection," or "ear infection" (the quotations are intentional, because most of us self-diagnose incorrectly), know that for the most part, these infections are viral and therefore cannot and should not be treated with antibiotics, which treat bacteria. When using antibiotics inappropriately, in addition to potential organ damage, there is risk of creating super bacteria or bacteria that becomes resistant to many antibiotics and can't be killed (e.g., MRSA-methicillin resistant *Staphylococcus aureus*). Antibiotic use should never be willy nilly and should be decided by a well-trained medical professional.

Drug Toxicity

35

Blood-Pressure Medications

"Water pills," or diuretics, are effective for releasing edema and sometimes for treating high blood pressure, but they have to be monitored closely to make sure they don't cause dehydration. Because they decrease the salt and water content in the urine and lower the volume of water in the body, problems can develop with the body's filtration system. Creatinine and BUN levels rise when this happens, which is why patients should check these levels regularly in their blood work when they are on diuretics like hydrochlorothiazide (HCTZ), furosemide (Lasix), and spironolactone (Aldactone). Sodium and potassium levels can be lowered, as well.

ACEIs are also very effective anti-hypertensive medications; however, they can affect the kidneys negatively, as well. (See Chapter 7)

Ultimately, each time these medications are considered and chosen for treatment, a reasonable risk-versus-benefit analysis has to be done to make sure the risk of renal damage, and other side effects, are worth the benefit of using them.

Illegal Drugs

Now onto the class of drugs that affects the kidneys in the most devastating ways—the "drug drugs" (e.g., cocaine, opioids, heroin, and amphetamines). For many reasons, none of us should take or even try any of these substances. One "hit" could be your last be it due to a heart attack, blood clots in your extremities or lungs, or an immediate stroke in the brain. The kidneys take an exceptional hit from illegal substances. Cocaine can cause acute kidney injury by either causing interstitial nephritis or tubular necrosis.[19] Evaluating any patient with a potential acute interstitial nephritis diagnosis warrants a complete review of the patient's drug history, if he or he has one. While the causes of cocaine-induced acute kidney injury (AKI) are multifactorial, interstitial nephritis specifically linked to cocaine use, though rare, deserves close clinical attention.

Illegal substances cause actual physiological effects, both direct and indirect to the kidneys, impacting overall kidney function. These pathological mechanisms may contribute to a variety of kidney conditions, including vasoconstriction (i.e., narrowing of blood vessels), renal cell damage from oxidative stress, acute kidney injury, chronic kidney disease, and end-stage renal disease. They also cause imbalances with acid, fluid, and electrolytes, like sodium, potassium, and magnesium in the body. Changes in kidney size and structure can occur, and hepatorenal syndrome (HRS), a type of acute renal dysfunction that also affects the liver, can be seen, as well.[20]

Rhabdomyolysis, or rhabdo, a condition involving damaged muscle breakdown and the release of muscle cell contents into the blood, is associated with the use of various illegal substances. Rhabdo can also be seen after strenuous exercise, such as after running a marathon, or

---

19 Tahmina Jahir et al., "Cocaine Hurts Your Kidneys Too: A Rare Case of Acute Interstitial Nephritis Caused by Cocaine Abuse," *Curēus* 12, no. 11 (2021), https://doi.org/10.7759/cureus.19236.

20 Editorial Staff, "Substance Misuse and the Kidneys: Effects of Drugs on the Kidneys," American Addiction Centers, last updated June 21, 2024, https://americanaddictioncenters.org/health-complications-addiction/renal-system.

trauma, like falling down a flight of stairs. Once it deposits into the organs, it can lead to serious consequences such as kidney damage and failure, irregular heart rhythms, seizures, and even death. In blood work, elevated creatine phosphokinase will be seen and, if the kidneys are affected, elevated creatinine and BUN levels as well. Urgent administration of IV fluids and oral rehydration, as well as correcting any electrolyte imbalances, will help prevent permanent damage.

Moral of the story: don't do drugs—for many reasons.

Tobacco and the Kidneys

Cigarette smoking is considered the most preventable risk factor for maintaining good health overall. Additionally, smoking reduces blood flow to vital organs like the kidneys, exacerbating existing kidney problems. Smoking harms nearly every organ of the body, according to the CDC. Unsurprisingly, smoking also plays a role in the progression of chronic kidney disease, first seen in a 1978 study.[21]

Nicotine causes increases in blood pressure and heart rate, which can both reduce blood flow to the kidneys. This triggers the production of angiotensin II, a hormone that narrows the blood vessels in the kidneys. Over time, this can damage the arterioles (small branches of the arteries) and lead to arteriosclerosis (thickening and hardening) of the renal arteries. Collectively, all of these changes enhance the loss of kidney function.

---

21 Davita.com, "Smoking and Chronic Kidney Disease CKD," accessed July 24, 2024, https://www.davita.com/education/ckd-life/lifestyle-changes/smoking-and-chronic -kidney-disease.

Smoking exposes the body to a range of harmful toxins beyond just tobacco. According to the American Association of Kidney Patients, studies have demonstrated that smoking can damage the kidneys, causing kidney disease to worsen and increasing the risk of proteinuria, or excessive protein in the urine.

The Multiple Risk Factor Intervention Trial was a research study that found that among men without kidney disease, smokers face an elevated risk of developing end-stage renal disease, with the risk climbing even higher for heavy smokers. Beyond its well-known links to heart disease, cancer, and other conditions, smoking has also been shown to contribute to renal failure in individuals without preexisting kidney disease.

Alcohol and the Kidneys

Little is known about the direct relationship between excessive alcohol or ethanol intake and kidney failure, other than the effects mentioned for illegal substances. However, alcohol abuse can lead to a myriad of health issues, often starting with liver disease that then progresses to kidney problems. Specifically, many kidney conditions are preceded by alcohol-related liver diseases. In these cases, while alcohol consumption is the underlying cause, the liver damage occurs before the kidney disease develops. A similar relationship exists with alcohol's impact on the heart. Excessive drinking is linked to cardiomyopathy and increased cardiac mortality risk. This alcohol-induced heart failure can consequently contribute to kidney dysfunction, as well.

Drug Toxicity

CHAPTER 5

Swelling

Swelling can occur on one or both sides of the body. It can be constant or intermittent. It can be due to something simple or open up a gamut of medical possibilities.

Kidney issues can lead to swelling if there is lack of blood flow or strain on the kidneys. Renal insufficiency or renal failure can cause decreased filtering through the small tubules inside the kidney, leading to increased protein in the blood and water being leaked out, thereby causing swelling. Other important organ-related dysfunction that can lead to swelling includes that of the thyroid or other endocrine glands, the heart (from heart failure or other cardiomyopathies), the liver, and a blood vessel (e.g., from venous insufficiency and disease). Standing for a prolonged amount of time, with gravity pulling everything down, or being stuck in an airplane for hours on end, exposed to atmospheric pressure, can do this, too.

So, what can you do? Limiting your salt intake is one thing. Avoid the French fries, salted pretzels, and potato chips. Salt and sodium are like magnets to water, causing swelling. Another trick is to get up and walk around every hour or so. When I was pregnant with each of my two babies, we traveled internationally. (If you've been pregnant, remember how much your legs looked like sausages?) I made sure to do calf stretches often when seated and get up every hour to do a lap in the aisles. I made sure to get a seat as close to the aisle as possible, to avoid getting on people's nerves.

If you're prone to edema, have your doctor prescribe medications or compression socks for you. You can also find compression socks or hose to wear during travel over-the-counter at a pharmacy or at a medical supply store. Medications, like furosemide (Lasix), spironolactone (Aldactone) or even hydrochlorothiazide can be prescribed for daily or intermittent use, if edema is a predictable issue, depending on the situation. Too much diuresis isn't a good thing, though, and can lead to dehydration, so use these medications with caution. Over-diuresing can also cause low sodium and potassium, and acid-base imbalances, which won't make you feel very well. In general, if you suffer from edema, drink at least 48 ounces of water daily, urinate often, and prop your legs up and rest when you can. It's all water.

The IV Hydration Trend

Used for wellness, self-care, and hydration treatment, this type of medical therapy is worth highlighting because it's been the talk of the town over the last couple of years. I also may be a little biased, because I provide this type of service in my wellness practice, as well. It's important, however, to make note that this may not be a safe option, especially in the regular doses of 500 ml, for patients with kidney disease who may be at risk of volume overload, or having too much fluid that won't move or becomes stagnant in or around the organs or blood vessels.

The intravenous (IV) hydration industry has seen a dramatic rise in popularity in recent years, expanding beyond its traditional medical uses to become a mainstream wellness trend. As people search for innovative ways to improve their health and address various concerns, IV hydration has emerged as a promising solution. Once confined to hospital settings, IV hydration has now expanded into wellness centers, spas, and even mobile clinics, allowing individuals to quickly and efficiently replenish essential nutrients, boost energy, and recover from the demands of modern life. This growing popularity of IV hydration reflects a broader shift in health care toward proactive wellness approaches, rather than reactive treatment.[22]

Recognizing that one-size-fits-all solutions fall short and that it's not for everyone, the IV hydration industry now offers personalized formulations tailored to each client's unique needs. It's also come under a lot of scrutiny in the medical community for being a quick fix for patients and not really providing any long-term benefits. If you become interested in getting these treatments for yourself, I would advise choosing a company run by a physician, and do your research first.

---

[22] American IV Association, "Navigating the Waves: Current Trends in the IV Hydration Space–American IV Association," accessed May 9, 2024, https://www.americaniv.com /navigating-the-waves-current-trends-in-the-iv-hydration-space.

PART 2

HEALTH CONDITIONS IMPACTING THE KIDNEYS

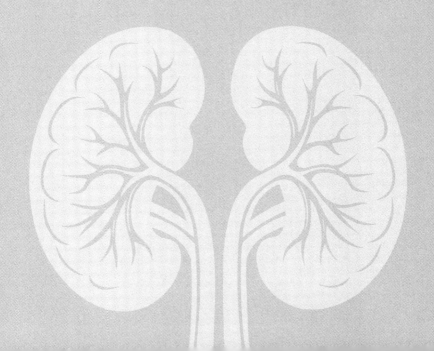

CHAPTER 6

Diabetes, or "the Sugars"

Almost everyone I know has a friend or loved one dealing with some type (1 or 2) of diabetes or has diabetes or prediabetes themselves. It unfortunately has become one of the most common, and most damaging, health conditions for Americans to date. The good news is we have made great advancements in both prevention and treatment of diabetes and are doing a better job at recognizing and treating diabetes-related complications.

Prediabetes

I'll touch on prediabetes briefly because it was always a topic of interest in my clinical practice. During most annual physical exams for adults above age 25, especially if there is obesity or a strong family history of diabetes, when blood work is done, either via finger stick or the vein, a hemoglobin A1c, or just A1c, is often checked. This is a measure of one's blood glucose control over three months' time. Normal levels are generally below a 5.7, and at or above 6.5 is considered diabetes. If a patient is between 5.7 and 6.4, there can be concern for prediabetes, which is one step away from being considered a diabetic. Fortunately, it can be treated with good nutrition, exercise, and lifestyle changes before ending up in the diabetic range. Some patients even begin taking metformin during the prediabetic stage to prevent becoming diabetic.

All in all, the goal is to prevent diabetes from happening or treating it as well as you can to prevent associated and likely irreversible kidney damage.

Type 2 Diabetes and Kidney Disease

Most diabetics will suffer from some form of kidney damage–whether it's from the sugar itself or potentially from the medications used to treat it. Over time, with diabetes comes high blood pressure, or the two conditions may have been diagnosed together and are being treated concurrently. Together, these health problems cause the large majority of kidney failure and the need for dialysis.

Regular insulin has been used for treating diabetes for decades. However, it hasn't been shown to actually help in preventing kidney failure. There has been concern about insulin causing long-term side effects, such as weight gain and wearing the pancreas out over time, which is counterproductive to the health of the kidney. The original drugs you may be familiar with: metformin (or Glucophage in the biguanide family), glipizide (or Glucotrol in the sulfonylurea family), and Actos (or pioglitazone in the thiazolidinedione family), unfortunately, have not been able to show evidence of preventing long-term kidney disease, except for controlling blood sugars alone. The newer medications, injections, and orals like Jardiance and Farxiga, have shown great statistics for prevention of cardiovascular disease, but not renal, specifically. There is still a lot of room for improvement.

The kidneys' tubules and filters are built to hold onto certain elements and filter through and let go of others. Depending on the health of the person and the strength of the internal system of their kidneys, the "walls" of the organs can become weak. When weakened, they leak. This is what too much glucose, otherwise known as sugar, does over time, because with poor health comes weakened walls of the kidneys, and the kidneys are the ones leaking glucose. Once the kidney becomes overwhelmed with a certain amount of glucose, the excess filters out first into the urine. This is why when you are being tested for diabetes, a doctor will use a dipstick to test if your urine is positive for glucose. Once the damage begins, in the blood work, the creatinine and BUN begin to rise, because creatinine, a waste product of the body, is normally removed from the body through the kidneys. Generally speaking, once creatinine increases to above 1.2 or 1.3 (depending on the gender of the patient and the lab being used), there is great concern for renal dysfunction occurring. Normal blood levels of creatinine are usually between 0.74 to 1.35 mg/dL for adult men and 0.59 to 1.04 mg/dL for adult women.[23]

Can diabetes be cured (and in essence, the renal disease associated with it)? I used to think the answer to

---

23 Mayo Clinic Staff, "Creatinine Test," Mayo Clinic, last modified February 9, 2023, https://www.mayoclinic.org/tests-procedures/creatinine-test/about/pac-20384646.

this was no. But, nowadays, with more research on healthy nutrition and eating habits, weight management, and physical activity (not to mention, bariatric surgery and the weight-loss injections), I'm rethinking that. Evidence now indicates that diabetes can be treated and cured completely, or be in what's called "remission."[24] That is incredible news.

Weight-Loss Drugs and the Kidneys

One of the goals of diabetic treatment is to prevent renal disease. Most newer treatments, like the GLP-1 drugs (glucagon-like peptide-1 receptor agonists), have great success in preventing the kidney damage that often accompanies diabetes, among other benefits like weight loss and cardiovascular improvements. You may have heard about these controversial injections, such as Ozempic (Wegovy) and Mounjaro (Zepbound), now being used for obesity. This generation of medications was actually created a while back, even before the weight-loss discussion. I recall talking to my patients about them when Victoza and Byetta hit the market almost 15 years ago. They were the first shots for diabetic control on the market with multiple health benefits, which later became known for having the wanted side effect of weight loss. Thus, the versions used solely for combating obesity were born.

---

24 Diabetes UK, "Weight Loss Can Put Type 2 Diabetes into Remission for at Least 5 Years, Direct Study Reveals," last updated February 26, 2024, https://www.diabetes.org .uk/about-us/news-and-views/weight-loss-can-put-type-2-diabetes-remission-least-five -years-reveal-latest-findings.

Since I'll be talking about several drugs in this chapter, I'm providing a chart that outlines each drug, its purpose, and its potential side effects. All GLP-1 injects affect the kidneys in the same way:

- **Pros:** Helps with glucose control and kidney disease prevention.

- **Cons:** Potential short-term kidney injury and worsening of chronic kidney disease.[25]

GLP-1 INJECTIONS

DRUG BRAND NAME	INTENDED USE (What It's Supposed to Help With)	POSSIBLE SIDE EFFECTS
Ozempic *chemical name:* semaglutide *dosage regimen:* weekly	Type 2 diabetes Used off-label for weight loss	Gastrointestinal issues, such as nausea, vomiting, diarrhea, and constipation
Wegovy *chemical name:* semaglutide *dosage regimen:* weekly	FDA-approved for weight loss only	Gastrointestinal issues, such as nausea, vomiting, diarrhea, and constipation
Victoza (no longer on the market) *chemical name:* exenatide *dosage regimen:* daily	Type 2 diabetes Was used off-label for weight loss	Potential increased risk of pancreatic cancer

---

25 Yuan Lin et al., "The Cardiovascular and Renal Effects of Glucagon-Like Peptide 1 Receptor Agonists in Patients with Advanced Diabetic Kidney Disease," *Cardiovascular Diabetology* 22, no. 1 (2023), https://doi.org/10.1186/s12933-023-01793-9.

Diabetes, or "the Sugars"

GLP-1 INJECTIONS

DRUG BRAND NAME	INTENDED USE (What It's Supposed to Help With)	POSSIBLE SIDE EFFECTS
Byetta (no longer on the market) *chemical name:* liraglutide *dosage regimen:* twice daily	Type 2 diabetes Was used off-label for weight loss	Potential increased risk of pancreatic cancer
Saxenda *chemical name:* liraglutide *dosage regimen:* weekly	Weight loss	Potential inflammation of the pancreas/ pancreatitis, gallbladder problems, kidney problems
Mounjaro *chemical name:* tirzepatide *dosage regimen:* weekly	GI effects and same as Saxenda and Byetta	GI effects and same as Saxenda and Byetta
Zepbound Tirzepatide *chemical name:* tirzepatide *dosage regimen:* weekly	Weight loss	GI effects and same as Saxenda and Byetta

Because obesity is often the root cause of most diseases that end up causing kidney failure, it is important to highlight the new innovations that are helping prevent obesity. With the rising popularity of weight-loss drug injections, I've received many questions from patients about the pros, cons, and costs. While Ozempic (sema-glutide) is perhaps the best known, it's technically an agent approved only for type 2 diabetes that has been used off-label for obesity. The same substance, semaglutide, is approved for use in obesity, but at a higher dose and under the brand name Wegovy. Alternatives are available, and

52   The **HEALTHY KIDNEY** Handbook

results will vary depending on the specific agent used and the individual.

Ultimately, I decided to try these new injections for myself. I am not a paid representative for, nor an advocate of, any of these medications; I'm here only to share my personal experience. In my discussions with patients about weight, I sometimes felt like an impostor. While I was overweight by medical standards, I fortunately had none of the underlying health problems. I wasn't on medications for blood pressure nor did I have diabetes, but I was counseling people to lose weight and eat better while not always following my own advice.

Since having children and turning 40, my metabolism, like many other women's, seems to have plummeted. I tried a number of older weight-loss medications, like phentermine and phendimetrazine, under the supervision of medical professionals. Each time, the efforts worked for a short while, particularly when I followed good portion control and practiced moderate exercise. Once the side effects (i.e., tachycardia, palpitations, mood changes, constipation) became intolerable, or I became tired or fearful of being on the medications too long, I'd stop and I would regain some of the weight.

When the newer subcutaneous injectable medications arrived on the scene, I was intrigued by their novel mode of action and seeming benefits. These medications, glucagon-like peptide-1 (GLP-1) receptor agonists, were first approved for type 2 diabetes, and it soon became apparent that patients were losing significant amounts of weight taking them, so manufacturers conducted further trials in obesity patients without type 2 diabetes.

The first of these, liraglutide, is injected daily and was first approved as Victoza for type 2 diabetes; it later received an additional approval for obesity, in December 2014, as Saxenda. Semaglutide, another of the new GLP-1 agonists, was first approved for type 2 diabetes as Ozempic but again was found to lead to substantial weight loss, so a subsequent approval of the drug for obesity, as Wegovy, came in June 2021. Semaglutide is injected once a week.

Semaglutide was branded a game changer when it was licensed for obesity because the mean weight loss seen in trials was around 15%, more than for any other drug and approaching what could be achieved with bariatric surgery, some doctors said.[26] These medications work in a different way from the older weight-loss drugs, which had focused on the use of amphetamines. The newer medications became very popular because treating obesity helps lower blood glucose, blood pressure, cholesterol, kidney disease risk, and other comorbidities that occur with diabetes. Plus, for most people, there were fewer side effects.

I first tried Saxenda when it arrived on the market, via some samples that our pharmaceutical representative brought, both out of curiosity and to see if it would help me lose the stubborn baby weight. I ended up stopping the daily injections after my second or third week because of nausea and vomiting. I took a break, got a prescription for anti-nausea medicine, and tried again because it did indeed decrease my appetite. However, when I took my prescription to the pharmacy, my insurance wouldn't

---

26 Matt Windsor, "Who Will Benefit from New 'Game-Changing' Weight-Loss Drug Semaglutide?" *UAB News*, April 9, 2021, https://www.uab.edu/news/research /item/11961-who-will-benefit-from-new-game-changing-weight-loss-drug-semaglutide.

cover it, which happens to doctors, too. Fast-forward to 2017-2018. The baby weight was still holding on despite lifestyle changes, diet, and exercising. The newer drug classes hit the market, and again we had samples from our reps. When our rep explained the potential for weight loss in patients without diabetes, I tried Ozempic off-label. Within the first two weeks, I noticed a 3- to- 5-pound weight loss.

When Ozempic was on backorder, I switched to a low dose of Mounjaro (tirzepatide), a new dual GLP-1 and glucose-dependent insulinotropic polypeptide (GIP) agonist, approved for type 2 diabetes last May, again using it off-label as a weekly injection, as it isn't currently approved for weight loss. However, it does produce significant weight loss and is awaiting approval for obesity.

SGLT2 Inhibitors

Sodium-glucose cotransporter-2 (SGLT2) inhibitors are the newest kids on the block, as of March 2013. They are a class of prescription medicines that are FDA-approved for use with diet and exercise to lower blood sugar in adults with type 2 diabetes. Medicines in the SGLT2 inhibitor class include canagliflozin, dapagliflozin, and empagliflozin.[27] They are quickly becoming just as important as ACEIs and ARBs (see page 69 for more on these two classes of medicine) in patients with chronic kidney disease. They cause great positive effects for preventing kidney disease

---

27 US Food and Drug Administration, "Sodium-Glucose Cotransporter-2 (SGLT2) Inhibitors," last modified August 20, 2018, https://www.fda.gov/drugs /postmarket-drug-safety-information-patients-and-providers/sodium-glucose -cotransporter-2-sglt2-inhibitors.

Diabetes, or "the Sugars"

and long-term complications from diabetes, but the biggest complication is the cost of these medications for patients. Once pharmaceutical and insurance companies help to make these drugs more affordable, more patients can afford them and benefit from them.

CHAPTER 7

Hypertension

To put it bluntly: check your blood pressure. Most national medical guidelines note that a normal blood pressure for an adult is anything around 120 on the top reading (called the systolic pressure) and 80 on the bottom reading (or diastolic pressure), usually written as 120/80. A pressure higher than this on a regular basis is now considered pre-hypertension. Hopefully, you and your doctor can talk and work on conservative measures to prevent higher levels and prevent having to take medicines. As we'll discuss below, hypertension can be caused by the kidney system and can be a consequence of kidney damage.

What Is Hypertension?

Hypertension is more commonly known as high blood pressure, or the force of blood pushing against artery walls. Arteries and other blood vessels supply blood from the heart to the other organs of the body, and veins and other blood vessels receive the same from the body's organs and return it to the heart. All of these blood vessels contain muscles that constrict, or tighten, and dilate, or relax, to control the flow of blood and fluid. When these muscles and vessels are too constricted or are constricted for too long, this can cause increased pressure and decreased blood flow. This is what is measured when you get your blood pressure checked with a cuff, or a sphygmomanometer, on a blood pressure monitor.

Your doctor listens to your heart beat, rate, and rhythm with a stethoscope, or a machine is recording the beat, to hear when the first beat drops (systole) and when the last beat is heard (diastole), while watching the numbers go up and then down. These two numbers make up your blood pressure. Most organizations follow the standard of the Eighth Joint National Committee (JNC 8), which noted that a blood pressure of 140/90 or less is normal.[28] That, of course, always depends on a patient's age and medical history. For those ages 60 and above, 150/90 or below is generally considered normal. If a patient has a history of cardiovascular disease, diabetes, or kidney disease, a lower blood pressure is desired, somewhere around 130–140/80–90.

Natural Remedies for High Blood Pressure

If your blood pressure is not well controlled, your risk for long-term kidney disease will be higher. Let's talk a little about natural remedies for high blood pressure.

---

28 Paul A. James et al., "2014 Evidence-Based Guideline for the Management of High Blood Pressure in Adults," *The Journal of the American Medical Association* 311, no. 5 (2014): 507, https://doi.org/10.1001/jama.2013.284427.

Vinegar

Have you heard about the use of apple cider vinegar to help treat high blood pressures? I first heard about vinegar in my third year in medical school in Charleston, SC. I was talking to a middle-aged patient with hypertension, whose mother and father also had high blood pressure and had for years believed that it could be cured or controlled with vinegar.

I was astounded at first to hear this, most of all because of the taste of vinegar and the thought that people were actually drinking it straight. The patient then clarified his family had taken over-the-counter vinegar tablets for years to treat hypertension. Some people swish and swallow it. But, instead of just discounting these beliefs, I researched them.

In history, vinegar's uses go way back to the times before Christ. Historical figures, including Hippocrates and Cleopatra, reportedly used it to clean wounds and make love potions, respectively. In the eighteenth century, it was used to clean hands while performing autopsies and then to treat ailments from rashes to abdominal pains. Today, it's being pushed as a cure for diabetes, obesity, and hypertension.

Let's look at the blood pressure theory. A 2001 of rats showed some lowering of systolic pressures, where vinegar seemed to prevent the action of a certain system in the kidney, thereby reducing blood pressure by about 20 mmHg points, or millimeters of pressure. But there's a catch: studies have never been conducted in humans. A 1999 study on nurses was done a little bit differently in that

Hypertension

the food studied wasn't vinegar alone but rather a vinegar-and-oil dressing.

Apparently, the nurses who ate salads with the particular dressing versus those who ate salads without it, did not have increased blood pressure or risk of heart disease. This doesn't mean, however, that they were healthier. There were other factors involved, like the mayonnaise content.

Vinegar does show some promise with blood sugars and the prevention of diabetes. In those who are at high risk for diabetes, studies have shown that ingesting vinegar can result in a modest decrease in glycemic control. Vinegar does this by increasing your body's response to the insulin you produce from your pancreas, especially if ingested about 30 minutes after meals.

So what does this mean? Unfortunately, the jury's still out on whether we can consistently say vinegar is the right thing to do for hypertension. However, it actually may prevent high blood sugar or diabetes in those at high risk. All in all, I always say the more prevention, the better. If you ever have any question about your numbers and your risk, discuss it with your doctor before making any decisions on your own that could cause more harm than good.

At one point, I tried ingesting vinegar myself for a couple of months (not for high blood pressure, just general health effects). Here's what I learned:

1. It tastes like vinegar: I tried my best to get used to the taste, but it's vinegar. I tried to shoot it like liquor once daily in the morning (bad for my acid reflux and apparently for your tooth enamel), diluting it in 8 ounces of water (it still made me shudder due to the vinegary taste). Now, recently, I've been doing more fruit-infused water to encourage more water intake. I'll add a splash of vinegar to that and won't notice it as much. So, it's a work in progress. Also, you're supposed to use a straw when you drink it to avoid damaging tooth enamel, so be careful.

2. I didn't lose weight: Play the loser music from *The Price Is Right* here. I was hopeful, but it didn't work. My male nurse, who is in his twenties, did notice about 10 pounds of weight loss after about a month of taking a teaspoon of vinegar daily, but he was also cutting back his calories and using other supplements. Oh well. Everyone's different.

3. I had a little more energy: I did notice and was very pleasantly surprised by the little jolt of energy I experienced about an hour after intake. I was able to cut back on my caffeine in the afternoon. That was a welcomed effect! So, I might keep a little in my life for that reason.

4. It didn't really work as a bowel cleanse: My bowel habits didn't change at all. I might have had some increased urination while using it, but that may have also been due to my increased water intake.

So, I won't discredit all of its proposed effects altogether, but at least I didn't experience any negative effects, other than the taste. Diluting it definitely helps. All in all, I give it a B-.

Cinnamon, Ginger, and Garlic

Cinnamon is thought to dilate and relax blood vessels, which would then decrease blood pressure. You can sprinkle the spice onto your food and drink, or take it in the form of a supplement. Studies have shown a significant decrease of both systolic and diastolic blood pressure by 6 and almost 4 points, respectively. This effect can be seen with consistent use of at least 12 weeks.[29]

Ginger has been used worldwide for hundreds of years for a number of health reasons. For years, I've encouraged patients to use it for morning sickness and nausea both in and out of pregnancy. Apparently, there is data that supports its use for blood pressure also. Studies have shown that those who consume 2 to 4 mg per day of ginger tend to have lower blood pressures.[30]

Another food I always get asked about is **garlic**. Like cinnamon, it also appears to dilate blood vessels and lower pressure. About a dozen research studies have shown a reduction of systolic and diastolic pressures of 8 and almost 5.5 points, respectively, when taking a daily dose of garlic for 2 to 24 weeks.[31]

These natural remedies and supplements should not be used instead of or along with your prescribed medications without first discussing with your doctor. Because they are not FDA-tested and approved for hypertension, and different brands may contain different amounts and other elements, they could cause counteracting or dangerous effects. However, for prevention of high blood pressure,

---

29 Seyed Mohammad Mousavi et al., "Anti-Hypertensive Effects of Cinnamon Supplementation in Adults: A Systematic Review and Dose-Response Meta-Analysis of Randomized Controlled Trials," *Critical Reviews in Food Science and Nutrition* 60, no. 18 (2020): 3144–54, doi:10.1080/10408398.2019.1678012.

30 Hossein Hasani et al., "Does Ginger Supplementation Lower Blood Pressure? A Systematic Review and Meta-Analysis of Clinical Trials." *Phytotherapy Research* 33, no. 6 (April 11, 2019): 1639–47, https://doi.org/10.1002/ptr.6362.

31 Karin Ried, "Garlic Lowers Blood Pressure in Hypertensive Subjects, Improves Arterial Stiffness and Gut Microbiota: A Review and Meta-Analysis," *Experimental and Therapeutic Medicine* 19, no. 2 (2019): 1472–1478, https://doi.org/10.3892 /etm.2019.8374; Healthline, "Does Garlic Cause or Treat High Blood Pressure?" April 24, 2024, https://www.healthline.com/nutrition/garlic-for-blood-pressure#bottom-line.

I would be comfortable with my healthy patients adding these foods to their regular intake.

Exercise and Blood Pressure

How much exercise is "enough" exercise? Most of us have a hard time keeping up and staying consistent, because... life. However, if you look it up, the national guidelines state that we should all aim for at least 150 minutes per week.[32] That equals 30 minutes for 5 days, or 50 minutes for 3 days—however you want to divide it up. The type of exercise that works well for both weight management and heart health is cardiovascular exercise–meaning the type that causes your heart rate to increase, your breathing to speed up a bit, and a little sweat on your brow to develop. Muscle resistance, through such activities as lifting weights, yoga, and Pilates, is great, but those usually do more for toning and muscle building than it does with keeping your heart healthy. Regular exercise is always better than remaining sedentary, especially for maintaining normal blood pressure.

Sodium in Food

We should all check labels (and learn how to read them, by the way) on the back of food items and note how much sodium is in one serving. We should also note that what's listed on the back is not what's in the total box or bag, it's

---

[32] Centers for Disease Control and Prevention, "Adult Activity: An Overview," CDC, last updated December 20, 2023, https://www.cdc.gov/physical-activity-basics/guidelines/adults.html.

what is in one serving, which could be one cup. To avoid eating too much sodium, try to avoid salty foods: potato chips, popcorn, canned foods, or packaged meats, for example. Instead of shaking salt on your meals, taste it first. You can remove your salt shaker from the table, as well, so it's not as easily accessible and reachable. Many of the combination seasons we love, for the likes of Cajun flavoring or meat seasoning mixes, honestly have too much salt in them (and I love those!). A good alternative to table salt for seasoning is the salt substitute version of seasoning. It contains more potassium than sodium, so it doesn't cause as much elevation in blood pressure. Go crazy on adding as much garlic, onion, cumin, pepper, cayenne, parsley, and other non-salty flavors to your foods without worrying about sodium.

Massage and Its Effect on Blood Pressure

I am a believer in physical touch, as a love language that heals many ailments. This is also true in medicine, in the form of acupressure, acupuncture, and massage therapy–whether Swedish, deep tissue, or other relaxing touch therapies. My husband, who has hypertension, and I (I don't have hypertension but have a family history of it) have been regular clients and advocates of scheduled massage treatments for the past decade or more. We get massages either at our home or at a spa on an average of every two to four weeks, mostly for relief from muscle and joint pain and stress, but I credit it as a reason my blood pressure has remained well-controlled for years. As mentioned, I don't have hypertension and hope to never have it, but as I get older, I believe massage therapy from a licensed massage therapist is part of my long-term preventive health care and wellness.

Studies have shown that both Swedish and deep tissue massage have shown moderate effects on blood pressure and heart rate after treatments. One study on deep tissue massage noted an average systolic pressure reduction of 10.4 mmHg, a diastolic pressure reduction of 5.3 mmHg, and an average heart rate reduction of 10.8 beats per minute (bpm).[33]

Not everyone is a hands-on person and not everyone likes to be touched, but you have the option of purchasing your own massage equipment (massage or stress balls, rollers, heated pads to go in your work chair or on car seats, leg compressors, etc.) to use at work or at home and possibly feel some of these great benefits on your own and on a daily basis.

Hypertensive Crisis/ Urgency/Emergency

Severe hypertension is associated with several risk factors, including advanced age, female gender, obesity, coronary artery disease, somatoform disorders (mental health problems that cause physical symptoms not caused by a medical condition), the use of multiple

---

[33] Wikipedia contributors, "Hypertensive Urgency," last modified April 7, 2024, https://en.wikipedia.org/wiki/Hypertensive_urgency.

blood pressure medications, and noncompliance with prescribed treatment. When huge elevations occur acutely, phenomena such as crises, urgencies, and emergencies can happen to patients.

When blood pressure is elevated, i,e., 180 mmHg systolic or 120 mmHg diastolic or higher, it's referred to as a **hypertensive crisis.** This condition, also known as malignant or accelerated hypertension, carries a high risk of complications. Patients experiencing a hypertensive crisis may not have any noticeable symptoms but are more likely to report headaches and dizziness compared to the general population. Other potential symptoms include visual blurriness or changes due to retinopathy, breathlessness from heart failure, and a general feeling of low energy from kidney failure. While many people with a hypertensive crisis have a history of elevated blood pressure, additional triggers can sometimes lead to a spike. There are several causes of hypertensive crises, including tumors, like pheochromocytomas.[34]

Hypertensive urgency describes a clinical scenario where blood pressure is significantly elevated (e.g., 220/125 mmHg) but the patient exhibits minimal or no symptoms and shows no signs of acute organ damage. In contrast, a hypertensive emergency involves severely high blood pressure accompanied by evidence of progressive damage to organs or bodily systems.

Hypertensive urgency is defined as severely high blood pressure without evidence of organ damage. Previously, "malignant hypertension" with advanced eye damage

---

[34] Wikipedia contributors, "Hypertensive Crisis," Wikipedia, June 18, 2024, https://en.wikipedia.org/wiki/Hypertensive_crisis.

was also included in this category. However, in 2018 new guidelines from European cardiovascular societies reclassified malignant hypertension as a **"hypertensive emergency"**—a condition requiring urgent treatment due to the risk of poor outcomes if left untreated.

In cases of hypertensive urgency, blood pressure should be lowered gradually to ≤160/≤100 mmHg over the course of hours to days. This can often be managed on an outpatient basis. However, the optimal rate of blood pressure reduction is unclear, as evidence is limited. Nonetheless, it is recommended that mean arterial pressure be lowered by no more than 25 to 30% within the first few hours.[35]

The medications that are most used for hypertensive urgencies are captopril, labetalol, amlodipine, felodipine, isradipine, and prazosin. We'll discuss these more in the next chapter, in terms of their class and actions on the kidneys. However, sublingual nifedipine is not recommended, as it can cause a rapid decrease in blood pressure, potentially leading to cerebral or cardiac ischemic events. Additionally, there is a lack of evidence supporting the benefits of nifedipine in controlling hypertension during these urgent situations.

When giving these acute medications, patients should be closely monitored for several hours to ensure blood pressure does not fall too rapidly. Aggressive dosing with intravenous or oral agents that lower blood pressure too quickly carries significant risk. Conversely, there is no evidence that failing to rapidly lower blood pressure

---

[35] Alan David Kaye et al., "The Effect of Deep-Tissue Massage Therapy on Blood Pressure and Heart Rate," *The Journal of Alternative and Complementary Medicine* 14, no. 2 (2008): 125–28, https://doi.org/10.1089/acm.2007.0665.

in a hypertensive urgency is associated with increased short-term risk for things, like stroke from hypotension, or low blood pressure.

The Classic Blood Pressure Meds

Diuretics

Hopefully, you don't end up with high blood pressure, or if you do, you're able to treat it with natural remedies. However, if it remains elevated despite your best efforts, medications are often prescribed. The tried-and-true meds, the diuretics, were the first to hit the scene. Chlorothiazide and chlorthalidone were the first to be used in European countries around the 1950s for hypertension. From these, derived hydrochlorothiazide, or HCTZ for short (brand name Maxzide), with which most of us are very familiar. We call them "water pills," or diuretics, because they diurese, or release water through the urine. This isn't the only way they help lower the blood pressure. The most important action that causes lower blood pressure is fixing the imbalance of sodium and potassium in the tubules of the kidneys. This is why we often see, potentially, lower potassium and sodium levels when they are checked in the bloodstream after starting them. These levels can be corrected by increasing dietary intake or taking over-the-counter or prescribed supplements, if needed.

You may have heard of Lasix, or furosemide, as well. It is also in the diuretic category of medications, but it works in a different way from the above medications. Lasix, and other diuretics like it, such as piretanide, bumetanide and torsemide, are called loop diuretics. They help block the receptors that absorb sodium chloride, thus reducing swelling because salt attracts water.

The ACEIs and ARBs

These magical medications have been on the market since around 1981. You may be familiar with the ACE inhibitors (angiotensin-converting enzyme inhibitors) by name: captopril (brand name Captopen), ramipril, enalapril (Vasotec), lisinopril (Zestril, Prinivil) and the like. Their "cousins," I like to call them, known as ARBs (angiotensin receptor blockers), were created shortly after the ACEIs and are usually used either in conjunction with the ACEIs in some cases, but more likely as an alternative to those that are allergic to the ACEIs.

I'm sure you've seen some pictures online or on social media like I have, of patients with swollen lips and faces, possibly from these medicines. It's a rare (about 0.3% of patients experience it), but very concerning and likely not fatal, side effect that can occur, called angioedema. African Americans appear to be more at risk for this condition by about five times the general population. This is thought to be related to a chemical found in the human body, called bradykinin. African American patients may be more sensitive to bradykinin, and the ACEIs tend to increase the amount found in the bloodstream.

Fortunately, angioedema is temporary, treatable, and reversible. ARBs, like losartan (Cozaar), olmesartan (Benicar), and valsartan (Diovan), bypass the system in the body that produces bradykinin, and don't usually cause angioedema. They are great "plan B's" to help with blood pressure, cardiac health, and kidney disease prevention or treatment for those that are allergic to the ACEIs.

Another, more common, side effect of ACEIs that ARBs generally don't have is a tickling cough. This is related to the same bradykinin process as the swelling, so thank goodness for the ARBs. Once the ACE is taken away, the cough usually dissipates and subsides.

Generally, the routine is to put a patient on one of these medications at a time, but in some instances, a patient is prescribed both an ACEI and an ARB for more prevention of nephropathy or congestive heart failure for those with a history. Oftentimes, these meds come in a one-pill combination with another medication, like hydrochlorothiazide, which is a diuretic, to give an even greater effect with lowering blood pressure and potentially lower extremity edema. However, you do want to be careful when taking the medications as a combination pill, because it can be more challenging to determine which medication may be causing a side effect and not making you feel good. You also want to monitor your labs closely, for things such as creatinine, potassium, and sodium levels, to make sure there are no imbalances.

Calcium-Channel Blockers

We can't forget about the classic calcium-channel blockers, like amlodipine (Norvasc), nifedipine (Procardia), verapamil (Verelan), and diltiazem (Cardizem). These medications have many uses now, but they are still used for blood pressure control and do a great job. Common side effects may include abdominal discomfort, nausea, and vomiting, but negative effects on the kidneys are rarely reported. They are great alternatives or add-ons for those with elevated blood pressure who can't tolerate some of the other medicines, or if they also have problems with chronic headaches, irregular heartbeats, menopausal hot flashes, insomnia, anxiety, angina (chest pain), headaches, and other medical conditions.

Beta Blockers

The other large group of antihypertensive drugs that is fairly safe for those with kidney problems is the beta blocker group. You may have heard of metoprolol (Lopressor, Toprol), carvedilol (Coreg), atenolol (Tenormin), and propranolol (Inderal) before. Other than being great anti-hypertensives and heart rate regulators, they are also used often for performance anxiety, tremors, palpitations, insomnia, hot flashes, migraine prevention, and other medical conditions.

Alpha Blockers

These medications include some of the original drugs we don't often use anymore because they've fallen out of popularity, but this class includes doxazosin (Cardura), tamsulosin (Flomax), and clonidine and prazosin (Minipress). I prescribed these frequently in practice to help with mood disorders, hot flashes, and insomnia in patients with psychiatric conditions or hormonal issues, because they help the blood vessels and body, literally, to relax. By blocking the alpha-1 or alpha-2 receptors in the vessels, they improve dilation. You may also recognize tamsulosin's name as a big help for those with enlarged prostates, or benign prostatic hyperplasia. The other medications in this class can be used for that also, along with lowering blood pressure.

The Atypicals

Did you know that Rogaine©, used for hair growth, contains one of the first widely used blood pressure medications—minoxidil. It is in the class of vasodilators, or vessel relaxants, like the medication hydralazine. You don't see these being prescribed as often as the above-mentioned medications, because they're older than most of them. Sildenafil, which is the main ingredient in many variations of medicines for erectile dysfunction, isn't necessarily classified as a blood pressure medication but can lower one's blood pressure. It contains phosphodiesterase inhibitors that cause this to happen. That's why we should always talk to patients about whether they suffer from blood pressure problems and take antihypertensives, because you'll want to be careful adding this on. A common side effect is a dramatic drop in blood pressure and a pounding headache as a result, in fact, because of this action.

CHAPTER 8

Glomerular Diseases

Kidney function can be impaired by various diseases and conditions that attack and damage the glomeruli—the tiny filtering units within the kidney where blood is cleaned. These glomerular diseases have many different causes.

Glomerulonephrosis is a disease that causes protein to spill through the filters of the kidney. Trauma, auto-immune disease, or external factors, like drugs and tobacco, cause protein to leak. Glomerulonephritis (GN), on the other hand, causes spilling of the blood. Think of issues that cause more infection than injury: viruses, bacteria, or parasites eat away at tissue, causing damage and bleeding into the urine.

When doctors check a patient's urine for clues (by urinalysis or urine dips), which include protein and red blood cell counts, these two disease types are what they're ruling out.

In pediatrics, we generally see more glomerulone-phrosis, because in many cases, patients are born with these diseases, or nephrotic syndromes. Syndromes such as focal segmental glomerulosclerosis (FSGS) and minimal change disease generally present in childhood and can cause symptoms like protein in the urine, swelling in the extremities (called edema), high levels of fats or cholesterol in the blood, and low levels of protein, or albumin, in the bloodstream. We still don't know what causes most of these cases.

Glomerulonephritis is known to be the complication of conditions, such as bacterial infections (namely streptococcal and staphylococcal), particularly when they go untreated, or autoimmune diseases, such as Wegener's granulomatosis and lupus (see the Autoimmune Diseases chapter). These diseases attack the tiny glomerular tubules of the kidneys (hence the name), which then empty their waste through the nephrons and filter them into the urine.

Focal Segmental Glomerulosclerosis

Focal segmental glomerulosclerosis (FSGS) is one in the group of glomerular diseases, characterized by scarring (sclerosis) in limited sections of the glomeruli. In FSGS, only a subset of the glomeruli are initially affected by this scarring. FSGS can occur in both children and adults, with a slightly higher prevalence in males and African Americans.

The tissue scarring associated with FSGS may occur due to an infection, a drug, or a systemic disease like diabetes, HIV, sickle cell disease, or lupus. FSGS can also develop secondary to another preexisting glomerular disease. FSGS is not caused by one disease, but can have many different underlying causes. Based on the underlying cause, FSGS is classified either as primary or secondary. The primary form of the disease arises spontaneously without an identifiable underlying cause. The secondary type is caused by another disease or exposure, such as viral infections (e.g., HIV) or certain drugs (e.g., anabolic steroids used for muscle growth, not the steroids prescribed for treatment).

In the early stages, FSGS may not produce any noticeable symptoms, but it normally causes a nephrotic syndrome. Some signs may include swelling in body parts like the legs, ankles, and around the eyes; weight gain due to extra fluid building in the body; foamy urine caused by high protein levels in the urine; high cholesterol; and low levels of protein in the blood (hypoalbuminemia).

To diagnose FSGS, a doctor will likely order several tests. A urine test measures protein and blood. A blood test can measure levels of protein, cholesterol, and waste products, indicating how well the kidneys are functioning. GFR also uses a blood sample, which will assess the kidneys' filtering capacity. Finally, a kidney biopsy, where a small tissue sample is taken and examined under a microscope, can confirm an FSGS diagnosis. Doctors may also recommend genetic testing to identify any inherited factors contributing to a kidney condition, which could guide the most appropriate treatment approach.

The specific treatment for FSGS will depend on the underlying cause. Since everyone's case is unique, a doctor will develop a personalized treatment plan tailored to individual needs. Typical treatments generally include:

- **ACEIs and ARBs**—These blood pressure medications can reduce protein loss and control hypertension.

- **Corticosteroids ("steroids") and immunosuppressive drugs**—These medications calm the overactive immune system to stop it from attacking the glomeruli.

- **Diuretics**—These help the body eliminate excess fluid and swelling, and can also lower blood pressure.

- **Dietary changes**—Reducing sodium and protein intake can lessen the workload on the kidneys.[36]

Minimal Change Disease

Many kidney diseases can impair kidney function by damaging the glomeruli. One such glomerular disease is minimal change disease (MCD).

MCD is a disorder in which very tiny changes are made to the glomeruli from damage, and so a powerful electron microscope has to be used instead of a regular microscope in order to see it. It is the most common cause of nephrotic syndrome in children.

Compared to other glomerular diseases, individuals with MCD tend to experience the signs and symptoms of nephrotic syndrome more rapidly. In adults, minimal change disease is usually secondary, meaning it is caused by another underlying disease or drug. Conversely, in children, MCD is usually primary or idiopathic, meaning the exact cause is unknown. If MCD is secondary, it may

---

[36] National Kidney Foundation, "Focal Segmental Glomerulosclerosis (FSGS)," September 29, 2023, https://www.kidney.org/atoz/content/focal.

be related to allergic reactions, use of certain NSAID pain-killers, tumors, or viral infections.[37]

Similar to other nephrotic syndromes, like FSGS, symptoms may not exist at all or classic ones, such as swelling, weight gain, foamy urine caused by high protein levels in the urine, high cholesterol, and low levels of protein in the blood (hypoalbuminemia), may occur. It is also diagnosed similarly, by either blood, urine, or kidney biopsy.

Due to treatments like corticosteroids or blood pressure medications, thankfully most children with minimal change disease usually fully recover. Rarely do patients suffer from chronic renal failure from this disease.

Post-infectious Glomerulonephritis

I've treated a lot of kids with this condition. It's a great one to be well-versed in and to remember with patients, because if you catch it, you can be a hero. Post-infectious glomerulonephritis is what happens to the kidneys if bacterial infections that we all deal with as children go unchecked and untreated.

Post-streptococcal glomerulonephritis (PIGN), the most common type of post-infectious glomerulone-phritis, is caused by the streptococcus (strep) bacteria. This condition most frequently affects children one to two weeks after a streptococcal throat infection, which we all know as "strep throat," and usually if it's left

---

[37] National Kidney Foundation, "Minimal Change Disease," May 9, 2024, https://www.kidney.org/atoz/content/minimal-change-disease.

Glomerular Diseases

undiagnosed and untreated. It also can occur if it's under-treated, meaning not treated with antibiotics (generally with one of the penicillins [Amoxicillin, Augmentin] or cephalosporins [Ceftin, Rocephin]) long enough. In my experience, this is often caused by patients feeling better after one or two days of treatment and then stopping their medication too early (of note, this also leads to resistant super bacteria). Less commonly, it can develop three to six weeks following a streptococcal skin infection. The 5 to 12 age group is the demographic most susceptible to contracting PIGN. After infections, the glomeruli become swollen and inflamed. The common symptoms are similar to those of other GN conditions.

For mild cases of PIGN, no treatment may be necessary. However, children are often advised to reduce their salt intake until the condition improves and the kidneys have healed. Medications may be prescribed to manage any symptoms, such as high blood pressure or swelling. Fortunately, most children fully recover their kidney function, though small amounts of blood may remain in the urine for several months.

CHAPTER 9

Autoimmune Diseases and the Kidney

Patients diagnosed with autoimmune diseases, or diseases where a body attacks its own self, generally have genetic predispositions to them. If their conditions are diagnosed early and managed well, hopefully lifelong and detrimental organ damage and complications can be prevented.

Systemic Lupus Erythematosus

Systemic lupus erythematosus, otherwise known as lupus or SLE, is one of the most common autoimmune diseases. It is a disease in which the immune system essentially attacks the body's different organ systems with its own antibodies and causes inflammation of the tissues of the organs. Organs that are affected include the kidneys, skin, joints, blood cells, brain, heart, and lungs.

African American patients are affected more than everyone else from this autoimmune disease. Not only are they three times more likely to develop lupus than White women, but often develop lupus at a younger age and experience faster disease progression and worse outcomes. You can often see the classic butterfly rash or hear of the joint pains and arthritis that can occur with lupus, but kidney disease is a common and unfortunate complication of this chronic disease. Lupus nephritis, or inflammation of the kidneys, leads to kidney damage. Renal failure is the most common cause of mortality for those with lupus.[38]

Lupus nephritis, a common complication of SLE, can manifest in various ways among different individuals. Common signs and symptoms include blood in the urine (hematuria); protein in the urine (proteinuria); swelling in the legs, ankles, and around the eyes; and weight gain, because of the inability of the kidneys to effectively remove fluid from the body, resulting in more weight and higher blood pressure. Glomerular disease can cause the glomeruli, the filtration units in the kidneys, to leak blood and protein into the urine, which will then be seen on urine testing. While the urine may appear pink or light brown, the blood cells are often only visible under a microscope. As previously mentioned, when there is leakage of protein from the blood into the urine, it can appear foamy.

SLE is typically treated with a combination of medications that help regulate the immune system. These include corticosteroids (such as prednisone) and antimalarial drugs. For patients with lupus nephritis, common treatments may include:

---

38 Lupus.org, "African Americans and Lupus," March 2013, https://www.lupus.org/s3fs -public/Doc%20-%20PDF/Ohio/African%20Americans%20and%20Lupus.pdf.

- **Corticosteroids:** These medications help calm the overactive immune system and stop it from attacking the kidneys.

- **Immunosuppressive drugs:** These work to suppress the immune system and reduce inflammation.

- **Monoclonal antibodies:** These are synthetic proteins that target and block specific immune system components.

- **ACEIs and ARBs:** These blood pressure medications can help reduce protein loss in the urine and control hypertension.

- **Diuretics:** These promote fluid elimination, which can lower blood pressure and alleviate swelling.

- **Dietary changes:** Reducing sodium and protein intake may help manage blood pressure and kidney function.[39]

Patients with lupus nephritis often undergo kidney transplantation. The anti-rejection medications prescribed to prevent the body from rejecting the new kidney are typically the same or similar to the drugs used to manage lupus. Interestingly, it is uncommon for lupus to recur in the transplanted kidney. In fact, lupus patients with new kidneys tend to fare just as well as other kidney transplant recipients.

---

[39] National Kidney Foundation, "Lupus and Kidney Disease (Lupus Nephritis)," May 21, 2024, https://www.kidney.org/atoz/content/lupus.

Rheumatoid Arthritis

Rheumatoid arthritis (RA) is an autoimmune disease that causes inflammation of the body's joints and soft tissue lining. It is related to a vasculitis, or inflamed blood vessels, and synovitis, or inflamed tissues, that can also attack the kidneys' filters. Patients with rheumatoid arthritis complain about the small joints of the hands and knees becoming deformed, swollen, and painful. Those with this autoimmune disease need to routinely monitor their kidney function and keep an eye on creatinine levels to avoid renal failure. The medications used to treat many autoimmune diseases, like methotrexate and steroids like prednisone, dexamethasone, and Solu-Medrol, should also be monitored for their potential effects on the organs.

Rheumatoid arthritis patients face an elevated risk of developing serious kidney disease, which in turn increases their likelihood of heart disease. In fact, individuals with RA have twice the average risk of cardiovascular complications. This compounded health burden can have grave consequences. Patients with RA face a 25% risk of developing kidney disease, which is significantly higher than the 20% risk for those without RA. However, the specific type of kidney disease is often unclear, as most RA patients with chronic kidney issues do not undergo a kidney biopsy. In the group of RA patients who did receive biopsies, a wide range of renal diseases were identified, including protein deposits that lead to kidney failure, accumulations of immune substances within the kidneys, and other conditions affecting the kidneys' tiny filtration mechanisms.[40]

While many rheumatoid arthritis medications are not directly toxic to the kidneys, certain treatments, similar to ones used for the other autoimmune diseases, can exacerbate issues if you have preexisting kidney disease.[41] Keeping RA well-controlled is important, because the better inflammation is managed, the more this will protect the kidneys in the long run.

Wegener's Granulomatosis

Wegener's granulomatosis, also called granulomatosis with polyangiitis (GPA), is an interesting and rare genetic condition that primarily affects the lungs and kidneys with vasculitis or inflamed blood vessels. When the blood vessels become inflamed, the walls become stretchier and can balloon out, causing aneurysms.[42] Vasculitis can narrow blood vessels to the point of complete blockage. This interruption of blood flow deprives organs of the oxygen and nutrients they need, leading to organ inflammation and damage.

When this disease is suspected, a biopsy of an affected area is often performed to confirm the presence of

---

40 L. J. Hickson et al., "Development of Reduced Kidney Function in Rheumatoid Arthritis," *American Journal of Kidney Diseases* 63, no. 2 (February 2014): 206–13, doi: 10.1053/j.ajkd.2013.08.010.

41 Arthritis.org, " Rheumatoid Arthritis and Your Kidneys Now!," accessed July 24, 2024, https://www.arthritis.org/health-wellness/about-arthritis/related-conditions/other -diseases/rheumatoid-arthritis-and-your-kidneys.

42 Cleveland Clinic, "Granulomatosis with Polyangiitis."

vasculitis. Biopsies are only recommended for organ sites with abnormal findings from examinations, lab tests, or imaging. Abnormal levels of tests, like ANCA (anti-neutrophil cytoplasmic antibodies) and other antibody tests, are markers of this disease. The diagnosis of GPA is also made based on the combination of symptoms and physical exam findings of affected tissue (such as skin, nasal membranes, sinuses, lungs, or kidneys). These same factors are critical in determining whether the disease is active or in remission after treatment.

Immunosuppressants or steroids are the mainstay of treatment of GPA, depending on the severity of disease. Examples of immunosuppressants are methotrexate, azathioprine, and mycophenolate mofetil, which can be used to prevent organ transplant rejection.

Goodpasture's Syndrome

For patients diagnosed with Goodpasture's Syndrome, the body mistakenly makes antibodies that attack and damage the lining of the lungs and kidneys. As a result, patients with this disease may experience fatigue, weakness, loss of appetite, and potentially severe complications.

Specifically, the disease can cause bleeding in the lungs, leading to coughing up blood, and can also inflame the kidneys, causing glomerulonephritis. The exact reason why the body starts attacking its own tissues is not fully understood, but potential triggers include viral lung infections, smoking, and exposure to organic solvents.

This syndrome is most common in people between 20 and 30 years old or after age 60, and it is more prevalent in men and Caucasians. It is not contagious. In some cases, similar symptoms may arise from other autoimmune disorders like lupus or Wegener's granulomatosis. It can cause severe, potentially fatal bleeding in the lungs, but this lung damage is typically not long-lasting. However, the disease often harms the kidneys, potentially leading to kidney failure that may require dialysis or a kidney transplant.

Similar to the other nephritis conditions, medications are prescribed to suppress the immune system and inhibit the production of harmful antibodies. Additional medications may be provided to manage fluid retention or high blood pressure. In some cases, a doctor may recommend a specialized blood filtration procedure called "plasmapheresis" to directly remove these harmful antibodies from your bloodstream. The body typically produces antibodies for a limited period, ranging from a few weeks to two years. Once antibody production ceases, lung-related issues should resolve. However, the kidneys may have sustained mild or severe damage. Despite this, the five-year survival rate is a relatively high 80%. Furthermore, less than 30% of people require long-term dialysis.[43]

---

[43] National Kidney Foundation, "Goodpasture's Syndrome," May 10, 2024, https://www.kidney.org/atoz/content/goodpasture.

Autoimmune Diseases and the Kidney

CHAPTER 10

Adrenal Gland Issues

The adrenal glands, which sit atop the kidneys, are critical to maintaining the body's equilibrium. These triangular-shaped organs produce hormones that control several important processes, including metabolism, blood pressure, immune reaction, and stress response. Adrenal tumors are atypical growths that appear in either the adrenal medulla (inner layer) or cortex (outer layer). Some of these tumors manifest as benign, but some may be malignant or release too many hormones, which may result in a myriad of bodily issues.

Adrenal Adenomas

Tumors and cancers can develop on the adrenal glands. Adenomas are benign tumors that are usually found incidentally on scans being done for another reason, or when hormone levels are checked and they are abnormal, followed by a tissue sampling, or biopsy for confirmation. They are noncancerous, for the most part.[44] They can be

---

44 Cleveland Clinic, "Adrenal Adenoma," accessed July 24, 2024, https://my.clevelandclinic.org/health/diseases/17769-adrenal-adenoma.

either functioning (active) or nonfunctioning (inactive). Functioning adrenal adenomas release excess adrenal hormones, potentially causing symptoms that require treatment. In contrast, nonfunctioning adrenal adenomas do not produce excess hormones and typically do not cause symptoms or require treatment. In fact, most adrenal adenomas are nonfunctioning.

While adrenal adenomas are generally not malignant, it is possible for a nonfunctioning adenoma to become functional over time. However, the development of cancer from an adrenal adenoma is rare. The most common cancerous tumor of the adrenal glands is adrenocortical carcinoma, which, like functioning adenomas, can secrete excess hormones and cause similar symptoms. Fortunately, adrenocortical carcinoma only affects about 1 in 1 million people, as the vast majority of adrenal tumors are benign.

A common endocrine condition called Cushing Syndrome is when an adenoma produces too much cortisol. While pituitary tumors are the most common cause, adrenal tumors can also lead to Cushing. Symptoms include weight gain (especially in the central abdomen), round face, and hump on the back between the shoulders (called the cortisol hump) which then leads to or is associated with high blood pressure, sexual dysfunction, and an increased risk of diabetes.

Another common adrenal gland condition is called primary aldosteronism, or Conn's syndrome. This disorder is characterized by an adenoma that produces too much aldosterone. Signs and symptoms include low potassium levels, high blood pressure, headaches, fatigue, and muscle weakness.

Treatment of adenomas either include surgical removal, or adrenalectomy and/or medications to reduce the increased production of hormones.

Pheochromocytoma

Not only is this one of my most favorite medical words to say, it's one of those unicorns we love to diagnose in medicine, meaning it's rare but very nice to find in order to help the patient. It's also very important, particularly for kidney health, because it can be the cause of very uncontrolled high blood pressure. Once a patient has been treated with at least three different blood pressure medications and the numbers are still above 160/90, for example, an alarm should go off for their doctors to check their blood and urine for signs of this tumor. This adrenal tumor produces what are called "catecholamines," hormones that can cause the blood pressure to rise. Levels of catecholamines are classically checked in the blood and urine and can diagnose pheo's, usually followed by abdomen CAT (CT) scans, magnetic resonance imaging (MRI), or positron emission tomography (PET) scans for confirmation.

It should be mentioned, however, that not all patients with this tumor will present with elevated blood pressure all of the time. In fact, individuals with a pheochromocytoma or paraganglioma may initially present with normal resting blood pressure but then experience sudden, severe spikes in blood pressure accompanied by symptoms like headaches, palpitations, paleness, and sweating.

Treatment usually includes surgery, radiation, chemotherapy, and other targeted therapies.

Adrenal Fatigue

This condition has been mentioned and highlighted a lot in the wellness and holistic medicine community. I recall being brought articles and lab order requests from my patient's holistic and naturalistic practitioners to add on to what we were doing for their general health on the traditional Western medicine side. I tend to think there can be a healthy balance of the two worlds working together for the betterment of patient health, if we both understand how to collaborate with the patient at the center and the helm.

That being said, I never quite understood the phenomenon of adrenal fatigue and how we are supposed to address it, treat it, and whether it was actually a "thing," but here's the research I've found. Based on Endocrine.org, there is no scientific evidence supporting it as a genuine medical condition. Doctors worry that misdiagnosis could prevent patients from receiving proper treatment for their actual symptoms. Also, the proposed treatments for adrenal fatigue lack approval from the FDA, the government agency responsible for regulating food and drugs, and are unlikely to be covered by insurance, potentially leaving patients with significant out-of-pocket costs.[45]

However, those of the adrenal fatigue theory believe that when the body faces excessive, prolonged stress, the adrenal glands become overwhelmed and unable to keep up with the body's demands. This, the theory argues, causes increased cortisol, leading to symptoms such as fatigue, sleep disturbances, and cravings for salt and sugar.

---

45 Endocrine Society, "Adrenal Fatigue," last updated January 25, 2022, https://www.endocrine.org/patient-engagement/endocrine-library/adrenal-fatigue.

There are no scientifically proven tests for adrenal fatigue, but I recall getting requests to check cortisol, testosterone, or other hormone levels, as well as to conduct adrenocorticotropic hormone (ACTH) stimulation tests. These tests, especially cortisol, should be checked at certain times of the day to be accurate; they are usually best fasting in the morning. Even if they are checked at the "right" time, they can be difficult to interpret. There is also no FDA-proven treatment for adrenal fatigue, but vitamins are often prescribed. Be sure to discuss this with your medical providers before spending the money to make the most well-informed decision.

Adrenal Insufficiency

This condition is the result of low cortisol, also called Addison's disease. It's the opposite of Cushing Syndrome, caused by adenomas. Common symptoms of Addison's disease include:[46]

- Darkened areas of skin
- Extreme loss of body water, also known as dehydration
- Severe fatigue
- Weight loss that doesn't happen on purpose
- Nausea, vomiting, or belly pain
- Lightheadedness or fainting
- Salt cravings
- Muscle or joint pains

---

[46] Mayo Clinic Staff, "Addison's Disease," Mayo Clinic, February 3, 2024, https://www .mayoclinic.org/diseases-conditions/addisons-disease/symptoms-causes/syc-20350293.

Adrenal Gland Issues

Treatment includes steroid treatments, like hydrocortisone, prednisolone, or dexamethasone, either to replace cortisol or stimulate cortisol production.

CHAPTER 11

Urinary Tract Infections

Although they're more directly related to the bladder, urinary tract infections, or UTIs, are a common topic of discussion around the subject of the kidneys. There has always been great debate about what causes UTIs and what treats them. Are they a natural occurrence? Are they caused by sexual intercourse? Do they happen to every woman after her menstrual cycle? Let's break it down.

First, let's think about the urinary tract itself. The urine exits the urethra, which connects to the bladder through valves, connected to each kidney by the ureters. There can be reflux into the bladder from the ureters with bacteria, which then develops into infections. Some common bacteria that cause UTIs include *Escherichia coli* (E. coli), Proteus, Klebsiella, and Citrobacter. In pregnancy, we often see GBS, or Group B Streptococcus, show up in the urine. It doesn't usually cause UTI symptoms but can cause irritation of the perineum—enough to contribute to premature contractions and labor. If these infections become severe enough, they can ascend up the ureters to the kidneys and cause true "kidney infections," or pyelonephritis.

When people have symptoms of UTIs, they will mention things like lower abdominal pain, side or flank pain, painful urination (dysuria), urinary frequency (polyuria) or hesitancy, strange odor or color to the urine, or even blood in the urine (hematuria). If severe, fever, nausea, or vomiting may be a complaint. My secret weapon, particularly in elderly patients who developed symptoms of delirium, confusion, or altered mental status, would be to check their urinalysis or urine dips. More often than not, they will have a positive urine for a UTI.

If a patient has mild symptoms and a positive urine test for an infection, and home remedies, such as cranberry juice, increased water intake, or over-the-counter medication such as Pyridium hasn't helped, a doctor can prescribe an antibiotic. The length of treatment depends on the severity of the case. Occasionally, if a patient has recurrent UTIs, a preventive or prophylactic dose of medicine, either daily or after a known trigger, like sexual intercourse, can be taken. This, of course, should always be discussed first with a medical provider.

Good hygiene is key for preventing infections to avoid affecting the kidneys. Avoiding holding your urine for more than four hours is advised. Wiping front to back to prevent stool from entering the urinary tract helps. Drinking more water than any other liquid is always important. Getting up after sex to urinate and wipe and maybe even washing down below can help, as well, for preventing UTIs, among other infections. Some prescribed medications, such as some of those used for diabetic medications, have UTIs listed as possible side effects, so pay attention if you've developed one "out of the blue" and you've started a new medication recently. Infections like bacterial vaginosis/ vaginitis and yeast infections can be triggered by similar things, but these would require a whole book on their own!

Pyelonephritis

When a UTI ascends and worsens to include systemic symptoms, such as fever, nausea, vomiting, and severe abdominal or back pain, pyelonephritis, which is an advanced and ascending bacterial kidney infection, can become a concern. Pyelonephritis is usually a reason for hospitalization, or at least emergency room care, involving IV antibiotics and fluids. Kidney stones can also become infected and present other issues.

If the infection in the kidneys remain uncontrolled or untreated, irreversible renal damage can occur. If the infection seeps into and spreads into the bloodstream, the patient can become septic with severe consequences, such as high fevers, low blood pressure (hypotension), confusion, coma, and unfortunately, death.

Vesicoureteral Reflux

Vesicoureteral reflux, or VUR, is a congenital condition when the "flaps" or valves inside the bladder where the ureters connect allow fluid and urine to flow the opposite way up the urinary system. This can be problematic and be the cause of frequent urinary tract infections. In infants and kids, if frequent UTIs are a problem before the age of two, VUR can be diagnosed by doing an ultrasound or a cystogram, where a catheter is inserted into the bladder with fluid to watch the flow of water with a radiology scan. This condition appears to affect female children more than male and can be corrected with medication, surgery, or implants.

Kidney Stones

Also known as nephrolithiasis, these collections of debris are severely painful and often difficult to prevent and treat. They are also the cause of many emergency room visits and pain pill prescriptions. These obstructions can occur anywhere up or down the urinary tract. If you review the anatomy section, remember the ureters start at the valves of the inside of the bladder and travel all the way up to the two kidneys. A stone can become lodged and stuck as it leaves the kidneys to attempt exiting the bladder, depending on its size.

Stones aren't actually made of stone, but rather are collections of either calcium oxalate (this is the most common), struvite, uric acid, or cystine. These elements are the "leftovers" from our digested food or elements found in the body. When they're not excreted in the urine, they can collect in the kidneys. Generally speaking, if stones are tiny, less than 5 mm, they can slide their way down the ureter and out of the bladder without much trouble. However, if there are multiple, or the size is more than 5 mm, the patient likely will need help and have significant pain.

Common symptoms can include excruciating back, side, or lower abdominal pain (depending on the location of the kidney stone), blood in the urine, painful urination, and more rarely, nausea, vomiting, or fever, especially if the stone is infected with bacteria. Most patients complain that the pain is akin to childbirth.

When patients come in with symptoms, doctors often start by doing a physical exam. During the exam, they might notice tenderness in the lower back area (around the ribs) or pain in the side or belly. Patients may also feel discomfort in the bladder area or just above it in the lower abdomen. To help figure out what's going on, doctors typically check the urine for signs of blood or infection. They may also use imaging tests like an ultrasound or an abdominal X-ray (called a KUB) to look at the kidneys, bladder, and surrounding areas, which helps determine the location and size of any stones that might be present.

Treatment focuses on easing the pain and helping the stone(s) pass from the body. Pain relief is important, as the pain from kidney stones can be very severe. Doctors may recommend strong anti-inflammatory medications, and sometimes short-term use of stronger painkillers like opioids. Most stones that are smaller than 5 mm can pass through the ureter (the tube connecting the kidneys to the bladder) on their own, though sometimes medications like tamsulosin (Flomax) are used to help relax and widen the ureter, making it easier for the stone to pass.

To catch the stone(s) once they've passed, patients may be asked to use a special "hat" with a strainer placed on the toilet. This helps catch the stone(s) so you can see they've been passed and collect them to bring to the lab for testing. Knowing what kind of stone you have can help guide dietary changes to prevent future stones, as some types are linked to certain foods.

Urinary Tract Infections

If your kidney stones are larger than 5 mm, you'll likely need a little extra help to get rid of them. One common treatment is shockwave lithotripsy (SWL), a noninvasive procedure that uses high-energy shock waves to break up the stone so it may pass more easily. This treatment works well for stones that are smaller than about 1 inch (2 cm) and doesn't require any cuts or incisions. Sometimes, doctors may insert a tube called a stent into your ureter (the tube connecting the kidney and bladder) to help the stone pieces pass more smoothly. The whole process typically takes about an hour, and you can usually go home the same day.

Another option is ureteroscopy, which is often used for stones stuck in the ureters (the tubes between the kidneys and bladder) but can also remove stones directly from the kidneys. This procedure is helpful for people who can't have shockwave lithotripsy, such as pregnant women, those who are very overweight, or people taking blood thinners. During ureteroscopy, a thin, flexible tube (called a ureteroscope) is used to find and remove the stone, and no cuts are made. You'll be asleep during the entire procedure, so it's painless.

If the stones are really large and can't be broken up with shock waves, surgery might be needed. One option is called percutaneous nephrolithotomy, where a small incision is made in the skin to insert a tube and remove the stone directly. Though this is more invasive, it's still less common today thanks to other treatment options. In rare cases, if the stone is extremely large or difficult to treat with other methods, traditional open surgery might be considered.

CHAPTER 12

COVID-19 and the Kidneys

Our world has never been the same since March 2020. We all lived through the confusion, chaos, and fear of hearing about this new infection caused by Coronavirus-19, watched it spread like wildfire, and watched the government and science world scramble to figure out what it was and how to protect us from it. We lost a lot of lives in the fight, and factions fought with each other on mask mandates, treatment, and whether vaccines were developed too quickly and without enough scientific evidence. Fortunately, four years later, we are in a more educated spot than we were then, and we continue to find out new information on a daily basis.

COVID-19 (Coronavirus disease of 2019) or SARS-CoV-2 (severe acute respiratory syndrome) can affect almost every part and organ of the body in a different way. I have never encountered another infection such as this in my medical career until now, that can for one patient cause simple and mild respiratory infection symptoms, and for another, cause stroke-like neurologic syndromes. For some, kidneys are greatly affected in negative ways.

Studies indicate over 30% of hospitalized COVID-19 patients experience kidney injury, and more than half of those in intensive care may require dialysis.[47] Early in the pandemic, some hospitals faced shortages of the machines and sterile fluids needed to perform dialysis on these patients.

Patients with severe COVID-19 can develop kidney damage, even if they had no prior kidney issues. Common signs of kidney problems in COVID-19 patients include high levels of protein or blood in the urine, as well as abnormal blood test results.

As it is with other organs, the way that the new coronavirus is able to infect and affect the kidneys is not yet well known. However, theories have begun to form with the cases we have witnessed so far. One theory is that the virus replicates within kidney cells, which have receptors that allow the virus to attach, invade, and make copies of itself. This can potentially damage kidney tissues. The same type of receptors are also present on cells in the lungs and heart, where the coronavirus has been found to cause injury.

The body's immune response to the coronavirus can be extreme in some people, leading to a dangerous condition called a cytokine storm. When this happens, the immune system sends a sudden, excessive rush of small proteins called cytokines into the body. These cytokines normally help the cells communicate as the immune system fights an infection. However, this sudden, large influx of

---

47 C. John Sperati, "Coronavirus: Kidney Damage Caused by COVID-19," Johns Hopkins Medicine, last updated March 1, 2022, https://www.hopkinsmedicine.org /health/conditions-and-diseases/coronavirus/coronavirus-kidney-damage-caused -by-covid19.

cytokines can cause severe, uncontrolled inflammation. In trying to eliminate the invading virus, this inflammatory reaction can end up destroying healthy tissue, including that of the kidneys.

Another theory has to do with the action of oxygen. The kidney issues observed in COVID-19 patients may stem from low blood oxygen levels, which often occur due to the pneumonia that accompanies severe cases of the disease.

Lastly, deep vein thrombosis or blood clots can occur in the extremities and organs for some COVID-19 patients. Because the kidneys act as filters, removing toxins, excess water, and waste products from the body, the formation of tiny blood clots triggered by COVID-19 may clog the smallest vessels and compromise kidney function.

The prognosis for patients with COVID-19–related kidney disease seems to depend on whether dialysis is required or not. Patients who do not require dialysis appear to improve better than those who do end up needing and receiving dialysis, particularly while in the hospital. Dr. C. John Sperati of Johns Hopkins hospital noted that among survivors of ICU-hospitalized patients with acute kidney injury requiring dialysis, about one-third fail to fully recover their kidney function by the time they are discharged from the hospital.[48]

As far as prevention is concerned, follow the same guidelines for kidney health, such as controlling blood pressure, eating a lower sodium diet, and avoiding toxins like tobacco and substances that injure the kidneys (see

---

48 D. Tuan, "Sperati Prevention and Management of Acute Renal Failure," April 12, 2010, https://www.slideshare.net/slideshow/02-sperati-prevention-and-management-of-acute-renal-failure-3704878/3704878.

Chapter 1). If you have a history of hypertension, taking your prescription medications correctly and regularly is also helpful in terms of preventing more damage if you are infected with COVID-19.

The Use of ACEIs and ARBs

Many news reports have questioned the safety of using certain prescription medications, such as ACEIs and ARBs, to manage high blood pressure during the pandemic due to concern that these medications' receptors make it easier for coronavirus to attach itself to and enter the body, making someone sick. Enzymes called ACE2 are in multiple organs of the body. It serves as the entry point for SARS-CoV-2, and is found in high levels noted in the gastrointestinal system, heart, lungs and kidneys. The concern surrounding the impact of ACEIs and ARBs on COVID-19 severity and mortality is twofold: One idea is that ACEIs might directly block ACE2, but this is unlikely because ACE2 works as a different kind of enzyme (a carboxypeptidase) and isn't affected by the ACE inhibitors typically prescribed. Another theory is that medications like ACEIs and ARBs could actually increase the amount of ACE2 in the body, which might make it easier for certain viruses to enter cells and multiply.

In response to all of this, the Council on Hypertension of the European Society of Cardiology strongly recommended that physicians and patients continue treatment with their usual anti-hypertensive therapy, stating "there is no clinical or scientific evidence to suggest that treatment with ACEIs or ARBs should be discontinued because of the COVID-19 infection."[49] On March 17, 2020, the American Heart Association, the Heart Failure Society of America, and the American College of Cardiology put out a joint statement advocating for patients to continue these medications as prescribed and that changes in medications in the setting of COVID-19 should be completed only after careful assessment by the patients' providers.[50]

---

[49] A. B. Patel and A. Verma, "COVID-19 and Angiotensin-Converting Enzyme Inhibitors and Angiotensin Receptor Blockers: What Is the Evidence?" *JAMA* 323, no. 18 (2020):1769–1770, doi:10.1001/jama.2020.4812.

[50] American College of Cardiology, "HFSA/ACC/AHA Statement Addresses Concerns Re: Using RAAS Antagonists in COVID-19," March 17, 2020, https://www.acc.org /Latest-in-Cardiology/Articles/2020/03/17/08/59/HFSA-ACC-AHA-Statement -Addresses-Concerns-Re-Using-RAAS-Antagonists-in-COVID-19.

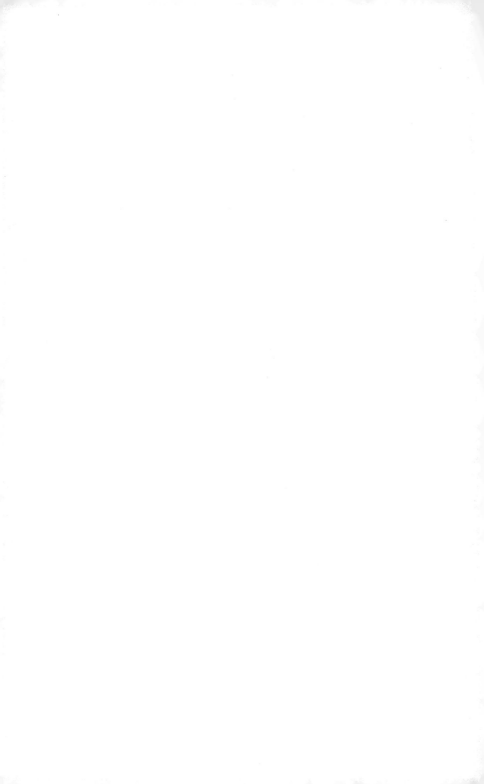

CHAPTER 13

HIV and Kidney Disease

Human immunodeficiency virus, or HIV, is a chronic infection that can lead to acquired immunodeficiency syndrome, or AIDs infections and other devastating complications. However, since the 1980s, great advancements in education, research, prevention, and treatment of this disease have increased the survival of many more affected patients than in the past.

Unfortunately, the disease can still affect multiple organ systems of the body, including the kidneys, and the most common syndrome associated with this is HIV-associated nephropathy (HIVAN). HIVAN is characterized by collapsing focal glomerulosclerosis (FSGS), tubular microcysts, and interstitial inflammation. Patients with HIV face heightened risks for kidney problems. This includes both sudden kidney injury and chronic kidney disease. The causes can stem from medication side effects, HIV-related kidney conditions, and immune system disorders. Additionally, as the HIV population ages, traditional risk factors like diabetes, high blood pressure, and obesity are leading to more comorbid kidney disease. Coinfection with hepatitis B or C also contributes to increased kidney disease in this patient group. Also, people of African descent have an 18-fold higher risk of developing HIVAN compared to those of European ancestry.[51]

Chronic kidney disease in people with HIV can show a wide range of patterns, often affecting both the tiny filtering units in the kidneys (called glomeruli) and the surrounding tissue. One major problem is HIV-associated nephropathy, but another condition called HIV-associated immune complex kidney disease (HIVICD) can also develop. HIVICD includes several different types of kidney diseases that can occur in people with HIV. These may include conditions like membranous nephropathy, membranoproliferative glomerulonephritis, and mesangial proliferative glomerulonephritis, as well as other diseases like IgA nephropathy and a lupus-like kidney condition called proliferative glomerulonephritis (some of these are reviewed in Chapter 8: Glomerulonephrosis and nephritis and Chapter 9: Autoimmune Diseases and the Kidneys).

Thankfully, the incidence of HIVAN has decreased with the use of effective combined antiretroviral therapies, and the incidence of end-stage renal disease in HIV positive individuals has decreased over time. However, people living with HIV are still 2 to 20 times more likely to develop end-stage renal disease versus those who do not have HIV. This increased risk is especially seen among African individuals, who have a sixfold higher risk of ESRD. While the incidence of ESRD due to HIV-associated nephropathy

---

[51] Saraladevi Naicker," HIV Nephropathy, a 'Vanishing' Disease in the Era of Antiretroviral Therapy?" *The Lancet*, accessed July 24, 2024, https://www.thelancet.com/campaigns /kidney/updates/hiv-nephropathy.

has stabilized somewhat, with around eight to nine hundred annual cases in the United States, the overall prevalence of ESRD in the HIV-positive population has risen. This is largely attributable to patients living longer and having increased longevity on combination antiretroviral therapy and a higher prevalence of kidney diseases, in general. As HIV-positive individuals live longer with continued treatment, a greater number are developing comorbid chronic kidney disease risk factors like diabetes and hypertension.

To prevent kidney failure and complications for this disease, national guidelines recommend regular screening for proteinuria and reduced kidney function in HIV-infected patients, starting at the time of HIV diagnosis. The screening interval depends on risk factors, which include Black race, HIV co-infection, low CD4 count, high viral load, and hypertension. The recent recommendation to start antiretroviral therapy immediately after HIV diagnosis may impact and, hopefully, decrease the prevalence of HIV-associated chronic kidney disease (CKD).[52]

---

52 A. C. Achhra et al., "Kidney Disease in Antiretroviral-Naïve HIV-Positive Adults with High CD4 Counts: Prevalence and Predictors of Kidney Disease at Enrolment In the INSIGHT Strategic Timing of Antiretroviral Treatment (START) Trial," *Supplements* 1, no.1 (2015): 55–63, https://pubmed.ncbi.nlm.nih.gov/25711324.

CHAPTER 14

Kidney Cysts and Polycystic Kidney Disease

Renal cysts are fluid-filled sacs that develop within the kidney. These cysts are categorized using a classification system based on the size and character of the cysts, called Bosniak, which helps determine their risk of being cancerous. While the majority of renal cysts are benign, simple cysts that can be monitored without intervention, some may be cancerous or suspicious for cancer and are often removed surgically through a procedure called nephrectomy. Numerous renal cysts are also seen in certain genetic kidney disorders, such as polycystic kidney disease and medullary sponge kidney, a condition developed at birth of small cysts on the tubules or the collecting ducts or channels of the kidneys.

The most complex cysts can be further evaluated with ultrasounds or contrast CT scans (a detailed X-ray imaging test to visualize the inside of your body). Depending on the level of complexity and concern, management of the cysts ranges from ignoring the cysts, scheduling follow-up, or performing a surgical excision and removal.

Polycystic Kidney Disease

PKD is the most common type of cystic kidney disease. It is genetic and broken up into two main types, based on genetics: **1.** autosomal recessive form (ARPKD) and **2.** autosomal dominant form (ADPKD). Autosomal recessive PKD is typically diagnosed in infants and young children, while the autosomal dominant form is most often identified in adulthood.

PKD impairs renal function and can progress to kidney failure. Additionally, it may trigger other complications, including high blood pressure, liver cysts, and issues with cerebral and cardiac blood vessels.

The signs and symptoms of autosomal dominant polycystic kidney disease, such as pain, high blood pressure, and kidney failure are also complications of the condition. In many cases, ADPKD does not cause any noticeable signs or symptoms until the kidney cysts grow to at least half an inch in size.

For autosomal recessive polycystic kidney disease, the early signs in the womb include enlarged kidneys and a smaller-than-average baby size, a condition known as growth failure. These early ARPKD signs are also considered complications of the disease. However, some people with ARPKD may not develop any symptoms until later in childhood or even adulthood.

While researchers have not yet discovered a way to prevent polycystic kidney disease, managing high blood pressure can help slow the progression of PKD-related complications, such as kidney damage. Aiming for a target blood pressure of less than 120/80 mmHg is recommended.

The sooner you know that you or your child has PKD, because of the genetic risk, the sooner you can keep the condition from getting worse. PKD is one of the most common genetic disorders, affecting about five hundred thousand people in the United States.[53] Getting tested if you or your child are at risk for PKD can help you take early action. If you know you're at risk for the disease, healthy lifestyle practices such as being active, reducing stress, and quitting smoking can help prevent or delay onset.

The course of polycystic kidney disease can vary dramatically, even among family members. While many individuals with PKD progress to end-stage kidney disease between ages 55 and 65, some experience only a mild form of the disease and never reach that advanced stage.[54] Other than preventing or treating kidney failure, complications of PKD include monitoring kidney cyst growth, high blood pressure, controlling pain, treating bladder or kidney infections, and watching for aneurysms (ballooning of blood vessel walls). If you have polycystic kidney disease and a family history of ruptured brain (intracranial) aneurysms, your doctor may recommend regular screening for intracranial aneurysms.

---

53 U.S. National Library of Medicine. Genetics home reference. Polycystic kidney disease website. Reviewed May 2014. Accessed December 7, 2016.

54 Mayo Clinic Staff, "Polycystic Kidney Disease," Mayo Clinic, accessed July 24, 2024, https://www.mayoclinic.org/diseases-conditions/polycystic-kidney-disease/diagnosis -treatment/drc-20352825.

CHAPTER 15

Kidney Cancers

Renal Cell Carcinoma

Renal cell cancer, also known as renal cell carcinoma, is the most common type of kidney cancer. While it is a serious disease, early detection and treatment significantly improve the chances of a full recovery. No matter the stage of diagnosis, there are steps patients can take to manage symptoms and feel better during the course of treatment.

Most renal cell carcinoma patients are between the ages of 50 and 70. The cancer typically begins as a single tumor in one kidney but can sometimes present as multiple tumors or affect both kidneys.

Doctors use a variety of treatment approaches for renal cell carcinoma, and researchers are continuously developing new options. It's important for patients to educate themselves about the disease and work closely with their healthcare team to determine the most appropriate treatment plan. It's generally seen as a mass on ultrasound on CT scan, which then needs to be followed up with testing.

The various tests to diagnose your condition may include:

- Urine tests
- Blood tests
- Biopsy to examine tissue samples
- Liver function tests to assess how well your liver is working
- Ultrasound imaging, which uses sound waves to create pictures of the organs inside your body
- CT scan
- Nephrectomy, a surgical procedure to remove part or all of a kidney, if a tumor has already been detected and needs to be checked for cancer.[55]

Treatment, like most cancerous tumors, usually involves surgical removal of the tumor, followed by chemotherapy, radiation, and long-term immunotherapy medications. If surgical removal isn't possible, percutaneous ablation (using a probe through the skin to the tumor while using imaging to guide and destroy the tumors with heat) may be an option.

Angiomyolipoma of the Kidneys

Angiomyolipoma is the most common benign tumor of the kidneys. Even though it is considered benign, sometimes

---

[55] Mary Jo DiLonardo, "Renal Cell Carcinoma," WebMD, March 24, 2024, https://www.webmd.com/cancer/renal-cell-carcinoma.

tumors can grow and cause bleeding in their large, dilated blood vessels (angio- means blood vessels) and impact the function of the kidneys.

The two most common causes or affiliated diseases with this cancer are a genetic disorder, called tuberous sclerosis, and a rare lung condition affecting women, called lymphangioleiomyomatosis. They are mostly seen in the kidney but can also be found in the liver or other organs, like the ovary, fallopian tube, spermatic cord, palate, and colon.[56] A ruptured angiomyolipoma, causing a retroperitoneal (meaning in the back of the abdominal cavity) hemorrhage, can lead to symptoms such as back pain, nausea, and vomiting. Long-term effects may include anemia, hypertension, and chronic kidney disease.

Treatment options include medications, surgical procedures, like embolization or creating a clot to prevent bleeding, and rarely, surgery. A treatment, called Everolimus, is US Food and Drug Administration-approved for the treatment of angiomyolipomas. Treatment should be considered for asymptomatic, growing tumors measuring larger than 3 cm in diameter.

Angiomyolipoma does not normally require surgery unless life-threatening bleeding is occurring. Some centers may perform preventative selective embolization of the angiomyolipoma if it is more than 4 cm in diameter, due to the risk of hemorrhage. Larger angiomyolipomas are treated by embolization, which reduces the risk of hemorrhage and can also shrink the lesion. A side effect of this treatment is called postembolization syndrome, or

---

56 Wikipedia contributors, "Angiomyolipoma," last modified July 21, 2024, https://en.wikipedia.org/wiki/Angiomyolipoma.

Kidney Cancers

after clots are formed, which can cause severe pain and fever, but this is easily managed and lasts only a few days.

Patients with tuberous sclerosis should undergo yearly renal scans, though those with very stable lesions may be monitored less frequently. Unfortunately, research in this area is lacking. Even if no angiomyolipoma is initially present, these tumors can develop at any life stage and grow rapidly. In tuberous sclerosis, multiple angiomyolipomas commonly affect each kidney. As a result, more than one surgical intervention may be required over a patient's lifetime. This is crucial, as kidney function can already be impaired (up to half the kidney may be lost before function loss is detectable), so preserving as much healthy kidney tissue as possible is vital when removing any lesions.

A ruptured aneurysm in an angiomyolipoma leads to blood loss that must be stopped (through embolization) and compensated for (through intravenous fluid replacement). Therefore, removal of the affected kidney (nephrectomy) is strongly discouraged, though it may occur if the emergency department is not knowledgeable about tuberous sclerosis.

PART 3

SPECIAL CIRCUMSTANCES

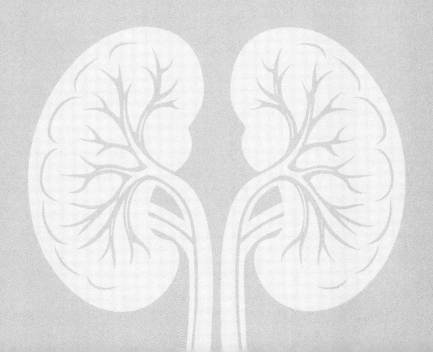

CHAPTER 16

Kidney Transplants

Once end-stage renal disease occurs and no other medication options are available, it's time to start planning for a transplant.

For patients with long-term kidney disease who are healthy enough to undergo major surgery, a kidney transplant is generally the optimal treatment, provided the potential benefits clearly outweigh the associated risks that may make it unsuitable for certain patients. The main disadvantages of a transplant include:[57]

- The surgery is a major operation, lasting two to four hours.
- The procedure can strain the heart and lungs.
- Patients must take powerful immunosuppressant medications afterward, which can lead to other serious medical problems.
- Some individuals experience psychological difficulties following the transplant.

Kidney transplants generally have very positive outcomes, with most patients experiencing many years

---

57 NHS, "Risks of a Kidney Transplant," accessed July 24, 2024, https://www.nhsbt.nhs .uk/organ-transplantation/kidney/benefits-and-risks-of-a-kidney-transplant/risks-of-a -kidney-transplant.

of good kidney function. While the risks of a transplant are typically much lower than those of remaining on dialysis, it's crucial to understand both the benefits and potential risks involved. Being informed about the transplant process will help you feel prepared to handle any issues that may arise after the procedure.

Before approving you for the transplant surgery, the transplant team will require you to undergo a comprehensive medical evaluation at the transplant center. This evaluation may include blood and tissue type testing, screening for HIV and hepatitis, prostate exams for men, mammograms and Pap smears for women, as well as heart, lung, kidney, liver, and colon exams.

Before receiving a kidney transplant, you will need to undergo tests to determine if the donor kidney is a compatible match for your body. For the transplant to be successful, the new kidney must closely resemble your existing organs and tissues, so that your immune system does not perceive it as a foreign threat and attack it.

Your immune system is designed to identify and eliminate anything foreign or harmful within your body, such as bacteria, viruses, or other potentially dangerous invaders. When a donor kidney is transplanted, your immune system will immediately recognize it as different from the rest of your body and attempt to attack it, just as it would a disease or infection. To reduce the risk of rejection, your transplant team will carefully select a donor whose blood type is compatible with your own. This helps ensure the new kidney is as close a match as possible, minimizing the chances of your immune system rejecting it.

If you have a living kidney donor, you can schedule the date of your transplant. However, if you are on the waiting list for a deceased donor kidney, you will receive an urgent phone call as soon as a kidney becomes available, instructing you to come to the hospital immediately. Once there, you will undergo a blood test to ensure your body will not have a negative reaction to the donor's blood. Provided the test results are satisfactory, the medical team will then prepare you for the transplant surgery. It's important to note that you may arrive at the hospital ready for your transplant, only to learn the donor kidney is not healthy enough for the procedure. While this can be discouraging, try to remain hopeful. Another suitable kidney could become available soon.

Once you've received your new kidney, which generally takes two to four hours in surgery, depending on if there are any complications, you'll spend some time recovering in the hospital. You will be under close monitoring to make sure your procedure went well. In some cases, your new kidney may begin producing urine immediately. However, with deceased donor kidneys, this process can take longer. If your kidney does not start working right away, you will need to continue dialysis until it does. Throughout your recovery, your transplant team will closely monitor you, adjusting your anti-rejection medications as needed to ensure your body accepts the new kidney. Once you're stable, you will be discharged home to follow up with your doctors in the clinic. Your surgical site typically requires about six weeks to fully heal. Immunosuppressant medications help prevent your body from rejecting the transplanted organ by suppressing the immune system's activity.

Kidney Transplants

Your body's immune system may reject a transplanted kidney because it recognizes the kidney's foreign proteins as a threat. This immune response, known as rejection, occurs when your body's defenses try to attack the new kidney. There are two main types of kidney rejection that can happen after a transplant:

- Acute rejection typically occurs within the first few months following the procedure. Out of 100 people who receive a kidney transplant, five to twenty will experience an acute rejection episode, and less than five will have an acute rejection that leads to complete failure of the new kidney.

- Chronic rejection develops gradually over the years after transplantation. In this case, the immune system's constant fight against the new kidney causes it to slowly stop functioning over time. Chronic rejection occurs more frequently than acute rejection in kidney recipients.

Hopefully, all goes well, the complications are minimal to none, and patients can return to their new normal as quickly as possible.

A Personal Account

A good friend and neighbor of mine is a kidney transplant survivor, and I wanted to document her thoughts on different parts of her journey. She is currently a married, African American woman, mother of a teenage son, in her forties, and works full time.

1. What do you remember about your time leading up to needing a transplant?

The cause of my end-stage renal disease was polycystic kidney disease (PKD), which is genetic. Of my grandfather's six children, four had kidney disease and three had transplants, including my mother and two of my uncles; their oldest sister had PKD but passed away from an associated complication (cerebral hemorrhage). I wasn't diagnosed until later, in 2010 about six months after my baby was born, when my doctor felt an abdominal mass on exam, and I almost immediately knew it was my kidney. We did an ultrasound, which confirmed the cysts, and we began our action plan. Thankfully, my kidney function was normal at that time. My primary care doctor referred me to a kidney doctor right off the bat to get a jump start on forming a relationship and staying on top of the disease. The first nephrologist didn't work out well, so I talked to my mom's nephrologist, who had transitioned from patient care to doing research, but he referred me to one of the practices with which he collaborated for research.

I started with once a year nephrologist visits, but when the early stages of ESRD began with increasing creatinine levels, the nephrologist and I, as the patient, worked together. I still had no symptoms at that time. Then, in 2014, my creatinine started increasing, and I began to have fatigue and feel exhausted all the time. At that point, we began talking about next steps. Our goal was to skip dialysis altogether and go straight to transplant, which I ultimately had in 2016. But before that, in 2015, I was referred to a surgical transplant team, took classes, and talked about donors. My brother thankfully decided to be my kidney donor, but because polycystic kidney disease is an autosomal dominant genetic process (meaning since our mom had the disease, we each had a 50% chance of having the disease), they needed to make sure he also didn't have PKD. It was a long testing process for him, so in the meantime, as my kidney function worsened, I had to start doing home peritoneal dialysis and had the surgery to place the abdominal port. Nurses had to do a home visit to make sure my home was an appropriate and sterile environment, with training for two weeks. I had a good experience with it and had to do dialysis 10 to 12 hours a night and did that for three months. Once we found out my brother was a match, we scheduled our surgeries for June 2016.

2. What was that process like with having your brother as your kidney donor?

My brother was a single dad at the time, so we had a very serious conversation about how this would affect his health and his life, too. We are nine years apart and he's the younger brother, so I was like his second mom his whole life. For him, there was no question that he would give me his kidney. So, I borrowed a kidney! We had surgery on the same day, but I'm not sure if we were in the same operating room or not, because I was sedated. Our mom was a nervous wreck with both of her babies on the table, but she had been through the same experience before with her own transplant. My mom's donor was her sister in 1998. All those in her family who received transplants were from living donors, which is atypical. One of my uncles' donors was a coworker, and my other uncle received a kidney from his stepdaughter. The whole family was there in the hospital when we had our surgeries. My brother was able to come home first, and I stayed in the hospital for three to four days to make sure I didn't have organ rejection or other complications. Generally, the stay is longer for most patients, but I was very determined to get up and move around and show the nurses that I was motivated and feeling well enough to go home.

3. What was the post-transplant process like after surgery?

I started my oral post-transplant regimen shortly after my surgery, and I now take one immunosuppressant daily. In the past, steroids were usually also part of the process, but thankfully, I don't have to take steroids. I have been able to avoid the side effects that can occur with steroids, like weight gain and infections. I also do IV infusions once a month, called belatacept (Nulojix), which can be very expensive. Thankfully, my insurance covers most of it.

4. What was the most challenging part of the transplant process?

Getting ready to have the conversation with your loved ones about having to have a transplant is extremely challenging. You have to manage both your and their emotions about it. Also, establishing the new normal, during and after your transplant is difficult, particularly since part of my journey has been during the Covid pandemic. My whole family had to mask for much longer than the mandates required to protect me from getting sick. My son, who was in middle school at the time, was more anxious (worried about me and feeling less socially engaged) and received occasional questions from his peers about why he was still masking. And my husband, who is also an educator, often had to explain that he was still masking for my safety. I still mask at work given my immunocompromised status, and we are all up to date with all of our vaccines. I'm even involved with a new RSV (respiratory syncytial virus) vaccine research study to help determine the dosing and effectiveness of the vaccine for immunocompromised patients.

5. Now that you're eight years out from the surgery, how are you and your donor doing?

We're both doing very well. I see my surgical transplant team now instead of my nephrologist, twice a year (once via telehealth, and once in person). I get my labs checked quarterly with my infusion, and I no longer have to have CT scans or imaging to monitor. I had an incisional hernia related to the transplant and had surgery recently to repair it; I had a hernia previously that was repaired when I had the surgery for the dialysis port. Having additional surgeries after your transplant is pretty typical for transplant patients, because of scar tissue and hernias that can occur afterwards. When I had my transplant, they also removed the dialysis port and did an appendectomy, as well, to remove my appendix, just in case it would later become a problem. I have had a conversation with my teenage son, but we have decided against doing genetic testing for PKD at this point because there's no cure or early treatment. For now, we just monitor his blood pressure and lab work to watch his kidneys. My words of wisdom for others going through this is to ask a lot of questions and don't go through this alone. As a community, we (Black folks) sometimes keep things too private, but there is a lot of support out there. Share what you're going through.

CHAPTER 17

Pregnancy and the Kidneys

Pregnant individuals with kidney failure face a significantly elevated risk of complications. Conversely, those who have undergone a prior kidney transplant generally have a more favorable prognosis.

Pregnancy triggers significant changes in the body, and the kidneys are no exception. During pregnancy, there is a notable increase in blood flow to the kidneys as well as a 50% rise in the glomerular filtration rate. This increased filtration capacity helps quickly remove wastes and toxins from the blood that could potentially harm the developing baby.

However, pregnancy can also place considerable strain on the kidneys, even for those with healthy kidney function. For individuals with preexisting kidney disease, the added demands of pregnancy may further compromise kidney function and worsen their condition. Reduced kidney function means waste products like urea can build up in the blood at higher levels.

Kidney disease can also impact the production of hormones that regulate blood pressure, putting pregnant women at heightened risk of developing high blood pressure and related complications. Overall, the kidneys undergo substantial adaptations during pregnancy, which can be challenging for those with underlying kidney issues.

Kidney failure can cause a range of distressing symptoms, such as swelling in the legs, ankles, or feet; itchy skin; headaches; muscle cramps; nausea or vomiting; reduced appetite; unintended weight loss; fatigue; weakness; difficulty sleeping; and anemia. Adhering to your prescribed treatment plan, whether that involves dialysis or a kidney transplant, can help manage or prevent many of these debilitating effects. Taking an active role in your care is crucial for maintaining your health and quality of life with kidney failure.[58]

Pregnant individuals with kidney failure face significantly higher risks of complications compared to those without kidney failure. Research indicates that this population has 2 to 10 times increased risk of adverse outcomes, including:

- High blood pressure due to pregnancy, including preeclampsia
- Miscarriage
- Preterm birth
- Low birth weight
- Small for gestational age
- Need for treatment in the neonatal intensive care unit
- Perinatal death

---

58 Jill Seladi-Schulman PhD, "What to Know about Kidney Failure in Pregnancy," *Healthline*, October 13, 2023, https://www.healthline.com/health/pregnancy/kidney-failure-in-pregnancy.

Given these substantial risks, it is crucial that anyone with kidney failure who is considering pregnancy consult closely with a healthcare professional. Increased monitoring and potential treatment adjustments will be necessary throughout the pregnancy to manage these elevated health risks.

Dialysis During Pregnancy

Pregnancy can significantly increase the demands on the kidneys of those with kidney failure who are undergoing dialysis. To keep up with this increased demand and protect the developing baby, dialysis treatment becomes more intensive during pregnancy. Dialysis may need to be increased to at least 36 hours per week, spread across five to six sessions.

This more frequent dialysis is crucial, as certain important nutrients like folic acid and protein can be lost through the dialysis process. Nutritional counseling is therefore essential to ensure the pregnant individual maintains adequate nutrition.

In general, a kidney transplant offers a better outlook for a healthy pregnancy compared to ongoing dialysis. As a result, doctors may recommend delaying pregnancy until after a kidney transplant can be performed.

Pregnancy outcomes have significantly improved for people with kidney failure who have received a kidney transplant. However, pregnant individuals on dialysis have also seen steady advancements in outcomes over the years.

One 2018 review found that live birth rates for those on dialysis increased from 37% in 1980 to 52% after 1990.

More recent studies have reported live birth rates of 80% or higher, potentially due to the use of more intensive dialysis regimens.[59]

A 2022 study on pregnancy outcomes in the dialysis population found a live birth rate of 71.4%, though preterm birth remained the most common complication. Other complications included small for gestational age (18.9%), miscarriage (16.9%), preeclampsia (11.9%), and high blood pressure (7.7%).[60]

Similarly, a 2022 review reported live birth rates between 72% to 93% for individuals with kidney transplants. A 2019 study in this population found a live birth rate of 72.9%, with preterm birth (43.1%), pregnancy-induced hypertension (24.1%), preeclampsia (21.5%), and miscarriage (15.4%) as the most frequent complications.[61]

Hypertension in Pregnancy

Because blood pressure is such an important topic on its own, I wanted to include some information on it during one of the most challenging times of life, too.

Gestational hypertension develops after 20 weeks of pregnancy. It usually causes a mild rise in blood pressure but in some cases can lead to severe hypertension and

---

[59] Jessica Tangren, Molly Nadel, and Michelle A. Hladunewich, "Pregnancy and End-Stage Renal Disease," *Blood Purification* 45, nos. 1–3 (2018): 194–200, https://doi.org/10.1159/000485157.

[60] H. Baouche et al., "Pregnancy in Women on Chronic Dialysis in the Last Decade (2010–2020): A Systematic Review," *Clinical Kidney Journal* 16, no. 1 (September 2022):138–50, doi: 10.1093/ckj/sfac204.

[61] S. Jesudason et al., "Parenthood with Kidney Failure: Answering Questions Patients Ask about Pregnancy," *Kidney International Reports* 7, no. 7 (April 2022):1477–92, doi: 10.1016/j.ekir.2022.04.081.

more serious complications like preeclampsia. Gestational hypertension typically goes away after the baby is born, but it can increase the risk of developing high blood pressure later in life.

During prenatal checkups, a healthcare provider will monitor blood pressure and urine to check for signs of gestational hypertension. They may also use ultrasound and fetal heart rate testing to monitor the baby's growth and health. A provider may ask a patient to check blood pressure at home and do kick counts to keep track of the baby's movements.

While we don't know how to prevent gestational hypertension, being at a healthy weight before pregnancy can lower risk. Even though gestational hypertension usually goes away after birth, those who developed it may be more likely to develop high blood pressure later on. Maintaining healthy habits like eating well, staying active, and reaching a healthy weight after pregnancy can help prevent future high blood pressure.

Preeclampsia/Eclampsia

Preeclampsia, a potentially life-threatening pregnancy complication, affects approximately 1 in 25 US pregnancies.[62] Although most people with preeclampsia deliver healthy babies, the condition can lead to serious health issues, including an increased risk of premature birth (before 37 weeks' gestation). Characterized by dangerously

---

[62] K. J. Chang, M. J. Seow, and K. H. Chen, "Preeclampsia: Recent Advances in Predicting, Preventing, and Managing the Maternal and Fetal Life-Threatening Condition," *International Journal of Environmental Research and Public Health* 20, no. 4 (February 8, 2023): 2994, doi: 10.3390/ijerph20042994.

high blood pressure and potential issues with the kidneys or liver, preeclampsia can develop after the twentieth week of pregnancy or in the postpartum period. This elevated pressure can strain the heart and cause complications during pregnancy.

If your healthcare provider determines you are at high risk for preeclampsia, they may recommend taking low-dose aspirin (also called "baby aspirin") to help reduce that risk. It's important that you take the aspirin exactly as prescribed—don't take it in higher doses or take it more often than your provider advises. Low-dose aspirin can be started anytime between 12 and 28 weeks of pregnancy, with the ideal time being before 16 weeks. Be sure to discuss the right course of action for you with your prenatal care provider.

Risk factors for preeclampsia include:

- Having had preeclampsia in a previous pregnancy
- Carrying multiple babies (twins, triplets, etc.)
- Having certain chronic health conditions like high blood pressure, diabetes, kidney disease, or an auto-immune disorder like lupus

There are other factors that can increase your risk of preeclampsia. Your provider may suggest low-dose aspirin for the following:

- Being a first-time mother or having not had a baby in over 10 years
- Having a BMI of 30 or higher (considered obese)
- Having a family history of preeclampsia

- Experiencing complications in a previous pregnancy, like a baby weighing less than 5 pounds 8 ounces
- Conceiving through in-vitro fertilization
- Being over the age of 35
- Being part of a population that experiences health disparities and racism, such as Black women
- Having a low socioeconomic status, which can limit access to quality healthcare[63]

---

63 "Preeclampsia," MarchofDimes.org, last updated April 2024, https://www.marchofdimes.org/find-support/topics/pregnancy/preeclampsia.

Q&A Section

As a family doctor, I've learned to be a person who answers the "dumb questions" that most people don't want to ask out loud. One of my favorite things to do is to educate the public about health issues, whether that be online, in articles, or via the media. So, in that same vein, I asked my Instagram followers what they wanted to know most about the kidney, and I'll rapid-fire answers to nine of the most popular questions I received:

1. How do you prevent kidney stones?

In general, staying hydrated with water to have regular urinary output is the way to go. If you have a history of kidney stones, called "nephrolithiasis" in the medical world, and know which type you have (calcium oxalate, which is the most common; struvite; uric acid; or cystine), you can avoid foods in the diet that cause those particular types of stones. Occasionally, doctors will prescribe preventive medications that can help prevent particular types of stones, as well.

2. Parsley tea as a detox. True or false?

I've never heard of this tactic, but I did a quick search online and saw claims about this being a drink that makes the urine more acidic, thereby causing toxins to flush out in the urine. Because it's not FDA approved or recommended, I'd take it to your doctor to discuss before trying it.

3. Can you inform people what an NSAID is and how it can cause kidneys to fail?

NSAIDs (non-steroidal anti-inflammatory drugs) are medicines like aspirin, ibuprofen, and naproxen. They help with fever, inflammation, and pain, but if taken too frequently or in high doses, they can cause kidney damage in the form of acute tubular necrosis and chronic renal failure.

4. What is the best type of water to drink for kidney health? Spring? Distilled, etc.?

I don't think that the type of water matters as much as the amount and regularity of water intake for kidney health.

5. How does IV contrast affect the kidney?

IV (intravenous) contrast is the dye that is used to help see things more clearly on radiology studies, like CT scans or MRIs. Scans can be non-contrast or with contrast. When IV dye is needed or requested, the patient's renal function and creatinine level is always in question, because if a patient has renal dysfunction, the dye can cause more damage (called contrast-induced nephropathy). Thankfully, this can be treated–either beforehand preventively, with IV fluids and N-acetylcysteine (NAC) and statins—or after an injury.

6. Can you live with only one kidney?

Yes, you can! Some people are born with one U-shaped kidney, called a unilateral renal agenesis, or the U-shaped uni-kidney, which is a rare condition. Or, some people donate a kidney to someone who needs it or have one partially or completely surgically removed due to trauma, cancer, or disease. They can live just as productively as those with two kidneys with close follow-up and monitoring with their doctors, of course.

7. When should someone start seeing a kidney doctor?

A patient should be referred to a kidney doctor, called a nephrologist, by their primary care providers when their hypertension is out of control, chronic renal failure gets to a moderate to severe level, or a mass is found on the adrenals or kidneys. Basically, the appropriate time would be any kidney-related health issue that can't be handled by your pediatrician, family doctor, or internal medicine doctor alone.

8. Are kidney infections caused by the same things that cause BV or yeast infections?

So, yes and no. Certainly, things like sexual intercourse and changes in urinary and bowel hygiene can cause all of the different "below the belt" infections. However, kidney or bladder infections are caused by different bacteria than bacterial vaginitis (BV, or vaginosis), and yeast infections are mostly caused by candida. They are, consequently, treated with different antibiotics or yeast medications. But, these infections can be triggered by sex, not cleaning properly after using the bathroom, or being immunocompromised or having chronic conditions, like diabetes. Side note: if you deal with recurrent BV and yeast, check your partner and see what's throwing your pH off. Men get these infections, too, and pass it on to their partners.

Q&A Section

9. I've had an ultrasound of the kidneys before, and my doctor said it showed hydronephrosis. What is that? Should I be worried?

No, hydronephrosis isn't usually worrisome, depending on the severity and the cause. It's basically a benign swelling of one or both kidneys, due to obstruction somewhere "upstream." We usually find it incidentally on ultrasounds, without the patient experiencing symptoms, but if it's severe, patients can have pain in the sides or back. If mild, as long as the cause is found, the dilation or swelling will resolve.

Conclusion

In conclusion, maintaining kidney health is essential for overall well-being, as the kidneys play a crucial role in filtering waste, balancing fluids, and regulating important bodily functions. Preventing kidney disease starts with a healthy lifestyle—eating a balanced diet, staying active, avoiding excessive use of harmful substances like alcohol and tobacco, and managing underlying health conditions such as diabetes and hypertension.

Regular check-ups and staying on top of any health concerns can help catch issues like kidney tumors or early signs of kidney disease before they become serious. For those already managing kidney conditions, working closely with healthcare providers to use medications appropriately and adopt any necessary treatments is key to slowing progression and protecting kidney function. By being proactive, you can help ensure your kidneys remain strong, functional, and ready to support your health for years to come.

Resources

American Heart Association (www.heart.org). Founded in 1924, the American Heart Association is dedicated to improving heart health and funding research to fight cardiovascular disease.

Centers for Disease Control and Prevention (www.cdc.gov). This national public agency works to promote public health, prevent the spread of disease, and prepare for domestic and international health threats.

Cleveland Clinic (my.clevelandclinic.org). Founded in 1921, this nonprofit academic health center and hospital is known for pioneering medical breakthroughs and is globally recognized for quality of care.

Endocrine Society (www.endocrine.org). This nonprofit organization is dedicated to promoting the prevention, diagnosis, and treatment of endocrine disorders.

National Kidney Foundation (www.kidney.org). This organization cites a mission to "eliminat[e] preventable kidney disease, accelerat[e] innovation for the dignity of the patient experience, and dismantl[e] structural inequities in kidney care, dialysis, and transplantation."

References

Achhra, A. C., A. Mocroft, M. J. Ross et al. "Kidney Disease in Antiretroviral-Naïve HIV-Positive Adults with High CD4 Counts: Prevalence and Predictors of Kidney Disease at Enrolment in the INSIGHT Strategic Timing of Antiretroviral Treatment (START) Trial." *Supplements* 1, no.1 (2015): 55–63. https://pubmed.ncbi.nlm.nih.gov/25711324.

Allarakha, Shaziya, MD. "What Are the 3 Types of Acute Renal Failure? Symptoms, Treatment." MedicineNet.com. Last updated January 5, 2022. https://www.medicinenet.com/what_are_the_3_types_of_acute_renal_failure/article.htm.

American Addiction Centers. "Substance Misuse and the Kidneys: Effects of Drugs on the Kidneys." Last updated June 21, 2024. https://americanaddictioncenters.org/health-complications-addiction/renal-system.

American College of Cardiology. "HFSA/ACC/AHA Statement Addresses Concerns Re: Using RAAS Antagonists in COVID-19." March 17, 2020. https://www.acc.org/Latest-in-Cardiology/Articles/2020/03/17/08/59/HFSA-ACC-AHA-Statement-Addresses-Concerns-Re-Using-RAAS-Antagonists-in-COVID-19.

American Heart Association. "How Much Sodium Should I Eat per Day?" Last updated January 5, 2024. https://www.heart.org/en/healthy-living/healthy-eating/eat-smart/sodium/how-much-sodium-should-i-eat-per-day.

American IV Association. "Navigating the Waves: Current Trends in the IV Hydration Space–American IV Association." Accessed

May 9, 2024. https://www.americaniv.com/navigating-the-waves-current-trends-in-the-iv-hydration-space.

"Angiomyolipoma." Wikipedia. Last modified July 21, 2024. https://en.wikipedia.org/wiki/Angiomyolipoma.

Arthritis Foundation. "Rheumatoid Arthritis and Your Kidneys Now!" Accessed July 24, 2024. https://www.arthritis.org/health-wellness/about-arthritis/related-conditions/other-diseases/rheumatoid-arthritis-and-your-kidneys.

Canadian Cancer Society. "Adrenal Gland Hormones." Accessed July 24, 2024. https://cancer.ca/en/cancer-information/cancer-types/adrenal-gland/what-is-adrenal-gland-cancer/adrenal-gland-hormones.

Carling Adrenal Center. "Adrenal Tumors Causing High Blood Pressure (Hypertension)." Adrenal.com. Accessed July 24, 2024. https://www.adrenal.com/adrenal-tumors/high-blood-pressure.

Centers for Disease Control and Prevention. "Adult Activity: An Overview." CDC. Last updated December 20, 2023. https://www.cdc.gov/physical-activity-basics/guidelines/adults.html.

Centers for Disease Control and Prevention. "Chronic Kidney Disease in the United States, 2021." Accessed July 24, 2024. https://nccd.cdc.gov/CKD/Documents/Chronic-Kidney-Disease-in-the-US-2021-h.pdf.

Centers for Disease Control and Prevention. "Chronic Kidney Disease in the United States, 2023." Accessed July 24, 2024. https://www.cdc.gov/kidney-disease/php/data-research.

Cleveland Clinic. "Adrenal Adenoma." Accessed July 24, 2024. https://my.clevelandclinic.org/health/diseases/17769-adrenal-adenoma.

Cleveland Clinic. "Granulomatosis with Polyangiitis (GPA, Formerly Called Wegener's)." Last updated July 16, 2019. https://my.clevelandclinic.org/health/diseases/4757-granulomatosis-with-polyangiitis-gpa-formerly-called-wegeners.

Cleveland Clinic. "Vesicoureteral Reflux." Last updated February 19, 2024. https://my.clevelandclinic.org/health/diseases/5995-vesicoureteral-reflux.

Davita.com. "Smoking and Chronic Kidney Disease CKD." Accessed July 24, 2024. https://www.davita.com/education/ ckd-life/lifestyle-changes/smoking-and-chronic-kidney-disease.

Diabetes UK. "Weight Loss Can Put Type 2 Diabetes into Remission for at Least 5 Years, Direct Study Reveals." Last updated February 26, 2024. https://www.diabetes.org.uk/ about-us/news-and-views/weight-loss-can-put-type-2-diabetes-remission-least-five-years-reveal-latest-findings.

DiLonardo, Mary Jo. "Renal Cell Carcinoma." WebMD. March 24, 2024. https://www.webmd.com/cancer/renal-cell-carcinoma.

Edwards, Jennifer M. "Is Renal Insufficiency the Same as Renal Failure?" *Healthline*. January 26, 2024. www.healthline.com/ health/kidney-health/renal-insufficiency-vs-renal -failure#renal-failure.

Endocrine Society. "Adrenal Fatigue." Last updated January 25, 2022. https://www.endocrine.org/patient-engagement /endocrine-library/adrenal-fatigue.

Endocrine Society. "Endocrine-Related Organs and Hormones." January 24, 2022. https://www.endocrine.org /patient-engagement/endocrine-library/hormones-and -endocrine-function/endocrine-related-organs-and-hormones.

Goyal, Amandeep, Austin S. Cusick, and Blair Thielemier. *ACE Inhibitors*. Treasure Island, FL: StatPearls Publishing, 2023. https://www.ncbi.nlm.nih.gov/books/NBK430896/figure /article-17070.image.f1.

Hasani, Hossein, Arman Arab, Amir Hadi, Makan Pourmasoumi, Abed Ghavami, and Maryam Miraghajani. "Does Ginger Supplementation Lower Blood Pressure? A Systematic Review and Meta-analysis of Clinical Trials." *Phytotherapy Research/ Phytotherapy Research* 33, no. 6 (April 11, 2019): 1639–47. https:// doi.org/10.1002/ptr.6362.

Hashmi, Muhammad F., Onecia Benjamin, and Sarah L. Lappin. *End-Stage Renal Disease*. Treasure Island, FL: StatPearls Publishing, 2023. https://www.ncbi.nlm.nih.gov/books /NBK499861.

"Hypertensive Crisis." Wikipedia. Last modified June 18, 2024. https://en.wikipedia.org/wiki/Hypertensive_crisis.

"Hypertensive Urgency." Wikipedia. Last modified April 7, 2024. https://en.wikipedia.org/wiki/Hypertensive_urgency.

Iadarola, Gian Maria, Elisa Giorda, Marco Borca, Daniela Morero, Savino Sciascia, and Dario Roccatello. "Is the Cost of the New Home Dialysis Techniques Still Advantageous Compared to In-center Hemodialysis? An Italian Single Center Analysis and Comparison with Experiences from Western Countries." *Frontiers in Medicine* 11 (March 11, 2024). https://doi.org/10.3389/fmed.2024.1345506.

Jahir, Tahmina, S. M. Sadaf Hossain, Ruby Risal, Marie Schmidt, Danilo Enriquez, and Mobasera Bagum. "Cocaine Hurts Your Kidneys Too: A Rare Case of Acute Interstitial Nephritis Caused by Cocaine Abuse." *Curēus* 12, no. 11 (2021). https://doi.org/10.7759/cureus.19236.

James, Paul A., Suzanne Oparil, Barry L. Carter, William C. Cushman, Cheryl Dennison-Himmelfarb, Joel Handler, Daniel T. Lackland et al. "2014 Evidence-Based Guideline for the Management of High Blood Pressure in Adults." *The Journal of the American Medical Association* 311, no. 5 (2014): 507. https://doi.org/10.1001/jama.2013.284427.

Jones, Taylor RD. "7 Nutritious Foods That Are High in Vitamin D." *Healthline.* Last updated July 6, 2023. https://www.healthline.com/nutrition/9-foods-high-in-vitamin-d#Vitamin-D-and-calcium.

Kaye, Alan David, Aaron J. Kaye, Jan Swinford, Amir Baluch, Brad A. Bawcom, Thomas J. Lambert, and Jason M. Hoover. "The Effect of Deep-Tissue Massage Therapy on Blood Pressure and Heart Rate." *The Journal of Alternative and Complementary Medicine/Journal of Alternative and Complementary Medicine* 14, no. 2 (2008): 125–28. https://doi.org/10.1089/acm.2007.0665.

Lin, Yuan, Te-Hsiung Wang, Ming-Lung Tsai, Victor Chien-Chia Wu, Chin-Ju Tseng, Ming-Shyan Lin, Yan-Rong Li et al. "The Cardiovascular and Renal Effects of Glucagon-like Peptide 1 Receptor Agonists in Patients with Advanced Diabetic Kidney

Disease." *Cardiovascular Diabetology* 22, no. 1 (2023). https://doi. org/10.1186/s12933-023-01793-9.

Maio, Giovanni. "The Metaphorical and Mythical Use of the Kidney in Antiquity." *American Journal of Nephrology* 19, no. 2 (1999): 101–6. https://doi.org/10.1159/000013434.

MarchofDimes.org. "Preeclampsia." Last updated April 2024. https://www.marchofdimes.org/find-support/topics/pregnancy/ preeclampsia.

Mayo Clinic. "Addison's Disease." February 3, 2024. https:// www.mayoclinic.org/diseases-conditions/addisons-disease/ symptoms-causes/syc-20350293.

Mayo Clinic. "Creatinine Test." Last updated February 9, 2023. https://www.mayoclinic.org/tests-procedures/creatinine-test/ about/pac-20384646.

Mayo Clinic. "Polycystic Kidney Disease." Accessed July 24, 2024. https://www.mayoclinic.org/diseases-conditions/polycystic- kidney-disease/diagnosis-treatment/drc-20352825.

MountSinai.org. "Creatinine Blood Test." Last modified August 20, 2023. https://www.mountsinai.org/health-library/tests /creatinine-blood-test.

Mousavi, Seyed Mohammad, Elmira Karimi, Maryam Hajishafiee, Alireza Milajerdi, Mohammad Reza Amini, and Ahmad Esmaillzadeh. "Anti-Hypertensive Effects of Cinnamon Supplementation in Adults: A Systematic Review and Dose- Response Meta-Analysis of Randomized Controlled Trials." *Critical Reviews in Food Science and Nutrition* 60, no. 18 (2020): 3144–54. https://pubmed.ncbi.nlm.nih.gov/31617744/.

Naicker, Saraladevi. "HIV Nephropathy, a 'Vanishing' Disease in the Era of Antiretroviral Therapy?" *The Lancet.* Accessed July 24, 2024. https://www.thelancet.com/campaigns/kidney/updates/ hiv-nephropathy.

National Institute of Diabetes and Digestive and Kidney Diseases. "Kidney Disease Statistics for the United States," March 5, 2024. https://www.niddk.nih.gov/health-information/health- statistics/kidney-disease.

National Kidney Foundation. "Focal Segmental Glomerulosclerosis (FSGS)." September 29, 2023. https://www.kidney.org/atoz/content/focal.

National Kidney Foundation. "Goodpasture's Syndrome." May 10, 2024. https://www.kidney.org/atoz/content/goodpasture.

National Kidney Foundation. "Lupus and Kidney Disease (Lupus Nephritis)." May 21, 2024. https://www.kidney.org/atoz/content/lupus.

National Kidney Foundation. "Minimal Change Disease." May 9, 2024. https://www.kidney.org/atoz/content/minimal-change-disease.

NHS. "Risks of a Kidney Transplant." Accessed July 24, 2024. https://www.nhsbt.nhs.uk/organ-transplantation/kidney/benefits-and-risks-of-a-kidney-transplant/risks-of-a-kidney-transplant.

Patel, Ankit B., and Ashish Verma. "COVID-19 and Angiotensin-Converting Enzyme Inhibitors and Angiotensin Receptor Blockers." *The Journal of the American Medical Association* 323, no. 18 (2020): 1769–1770. https://doi.org/10.1001/jama.2020.4812.

Ried, Karin. "Garlic Lowers Blood Pressure in Hypertensive Subjects, Improves Arterial Stiffness and Gut Microbiota: A Review and Meta-Analysis." *Experimental and Therapeutic Medicine*, 19, no. 2 (2019): 1472-1478. https://doi.org/10.3892/etm.2019.8374.

Seladi-Schulman, Jill, PhD. "What to Know about Kidney Failure in Pregnancy." *Healthline*. October 13, 2023. https://www.healthline.com/health/pregnancy/kidney-failure-in-pregnancy.

Sperati, C. John. "Coronavirus: Kidney Damage Caused by COVID-19." Johns Hopkins Medicine. Last updated March 1, 2022. https://www.hopkinsmedicine.org/health/conditions-and-diseases/coronavirus/coronavirus-kidney-damage-caused-by-covid19.

Texas Kidney Institute. "The 5 Stages of Kidney Disease, Explained." December 8, 2020. https://texaskidneyinstitute.com/the-5-stages-of-kidney-disease-explained.

Tkacs, Nancy C., Linda L. Herrmann, and Randall L. Johnson. *Advanced Physiology and Pathophysiology: Essentials for Clinical Practice.* Springer Publishing Company, Manhattan, NYC, 2020.

US Department of Health and Human Services. *Physical Activity Guidelines for Americans, 2nd Edition.* Washington, DC: US Department of Health and Human Services, 2018. https://health.gov/sites/default/files/2019-09/Physical_Activity_Guidelines_2nd_edition.pdf.

US Food and Drug Administration. "Sodium-Glucose Cotransporter-2 (SGLT2) Inhibitors." Last modified August 20, 2018. https://www.fda.gov/drugs/postmarket-drug-safety-information-patients-and-providers/sodium-glucose-cotransporter-2-sglt2-inhibitors.

US National Library of Medicine. Genetics Home Reference. Polycystic Kidney Disease Website. Reviewed May 2014. Accessed December 7, 2016.

Whitbourne, Kathryn. "Kidney Stone Surgery: Types, Risks, and Recovery." WebMD. June 7, 2024. https://www.webmd.com/kidney-stones/surgery-for-kidney-stone.

Windsor, Matt. "Who Will Benefit from New 'Game-Changing' Weight-Loss Drug Semaglutide?" *UAB News.* April 9, 2021. https://www.uab.edu/news/research/item/11961-who-will-benefit-from-new-game-changing-weight-loss-drug-semaglutide.

Index

A

accelerated hypertension. *See* hypertensive crisis
acetaminophen (Tylenol), 33
Actos, 48
acute kidney injury (AKI), 37
acute rejection, 122
acute renal dysfunction, 37
acute renal failure (ARF), 24
Addison's disease. *See* adrenal insufficiency
adrenal adenomas, 87–89
  Conn's syndrome, 88
  Cushing syndrome, 88
  pheochromocytoma, 89
adrenal fatigue, 90–91
adrenal gland issues, 87–92
  adrenal adenomas, 87–89
  adrenal fatigue, 90–91
  adrenal insufficiency, 91–92
adrenal glands, 3, 9
adrenal insufficiency, 91–92
adrenaline, 9
adrenaline-related hormones, 9

adrenocorticotropic hormone (ACTH) stimulation tests, 91
alcohol and kidneys, 39
aldosterone, 10
alpha blockers, 71–72
aminoglycoside class of antibiotics, 35
amlodipine (Norvasc), 67, 70
amphetamines, 54
androgens, 9–10
anemia, 27
aneurysms (ballooning of blood vessel walls), 83, 111
  intracranial, 111
angiomyolipoma, 114–116
angiotensin II, 38
angiotensin receptor blockers (ARBs), 11, 75–76, 81, 102–103
angiotensin-converting enzyme (ACE), 11
angiotensin-converting enzyme inhibitors (ACEIs), 69, 75–76, 81, 102–103
antibiotics, 34–35
  aminoglycoside class of, 35
  cephalosporin class of, 34

anti-hypertensive
medications,36
anti-hypertensive therapy, 102
antineutrophil cytoplasmic
antibodies (ANCA), 84
arterioles, 38
arteriosclerosis, 38
arteriovenous (AV) fistulas, 28
atenolol (Tenormin), 71
atypicals, 72
autoimmune diseases
and kidney, 79–85. *See
also* systemic lupus
erythematosus (SLE)
Goodpasture's syndrome,
84–85
rheumatoid arthritis (RA),
82–83
Wegener's granulomatosis,
83–84
automated peritoneal dialysis
(APD), 32
autosomal dominant form
(ADPKD), 110
autosomal recessive form
(ARPKD), 110
azathioprine, 84

B
baby aspirin, 134
belatacept (Nulojix), 123
beta blockers, 71
blood-pressure medications, 36
blood pressure, natural
remedies for, 58–68. *See also*
classic blood pressure meds
cinnamon, 61–63

exercise, 63
garlic, 61–63
ginger, 61–63
hypertensive urgency, 66
massage, 64–65
sodium in food, 63–64
vinegar, 59–61
blood urea nitrogen (BUN), 15,
23
BUN to creatinine ratio, 26
Byetta, 52

C
calcium-channel blockers,
70–71
canagliflozin, 55
cancer in kidneys, 113–116
angiomyolipoma, 114–116
renal cell carcinoma, 113–114
captopril, 67, 69
carvedilol (Coreg), 71
catecholamines, 89
ceftriaxone (Rocephin), 34
cefuroxime (Ceftin), 34
cellulitis, 34
Centers for Disease Control
(CDC), vii, 1
cephalexin (Keflex), 34
cephalosporins [Ceftin,
Rocephin], 34, 78
chronic kidney disease (CKD),
1, 18, 106–107
racial prevalence, 1–2
Stage 1 or 2, 27
Stage 3, 27
Stage 4, 28
Stage 5, 28

154   The **HEALTHY KIDNEY** Handbook

stages, 27–28
chronic rejection, 122
chronic renal failure (CRF), 24
cigarette smoking and kidney, 38
cinnamon, for high blood pressure, 61–63
ciprofloxacin, 34
classic blood pressure meds, 68–69
    diuretics, 68–69
clonidine, 71
cocaine, 37
Conn's syndrome, 88
contrast-induced nephropathy, 138
corticosteroids, 76, 81
cortisol, 10
COVID-19 and kidney, 99–103
    ACEIs for, 102–103
    ARBs for, 102–103
    cytokine storm, 100
creatinine (Cr) level, 15, 23
Cushing syndrome, 88, 91
cysts, 109–111
    kidney cysts and polycystic kidney disease, 109–111
cytokine storm, 100

D
dapagliflozin, 55
dexamethasone, 92
diabetes (the Sugars), 3, 47–56. *See also* weight-loss drugs and kidney
    prediabetes, 47–48

type 2 diabetes and kidney disease, 48–50
dialysis, 2, 28–30
    arteriovenous (AV) fistulas, 28
    during pregnancy, 131–132
    hemodialysis vs. peritoneal dialysis, 30–32
        cons, 30–32
        pros, 30–32
    peritoneal dialysis, 29
dietary changes, 76
1,25-dihydroxyvitamin D (calcitriol), 19
diltiazem (Cardizem), 70
diuretics, 68–69, 76, 81
doxazosin (Cardura), 71
drug toxicity, 33–39
    antibiotics, 34–35
    illegal drugs, 36–38
dysuria (painful urination), 25, 94

E
empagliflozin, 55
enalapril (Vasotec), 69
end-stage renal disease (ESRD), 23
epinephrine, 9
Epo, 27
erythropoiesis, 27
estrogen, 9–10
exercise and blood pressure, 63

F
Farxiga, 49
felodipine, 67

floroquinolones, 34
focal glomerulosclerosis
(FSGS), 105
focal segmental
glomerulosclerosis (FSGS),
73–76
treatments, 75
ACEIs, 75
ARBs, 75
corticosteroids, 76
dietary changes, 76
diuretics, 76
furosemide (Lasix), 36, 42

G

garlic, for high blood pressure,
61–63
gestational hypertension, 132
Gibson, Keisha L., ix
ginger, for high blood pressure,
61–63
glipizide, 48
glomerular diseases, 73–78
focal segmental
glomerulosclerosis
(FSGS), 74–76
minimal change disease
(MCD), 76–77
post-infectious
glomerulonephritis, 77–78
glomerular filtration rate
(GFR), 23
glomeruli, 106
glomerulonephritis (GN), 73, 77
GLP-1 drugs (glucagon-like
peptide-1 receptor agonists),
50–53

Byetta, 52
cons, 51
injections, 51–52
Mounjaro, 50, 52
Ozempic, 50–51
pros, 51
Saxenda, 52
Wegovy, 51
Zepbound Tirzepatide, 52
glucocorticoids and sex
hormones, 10
glycoprotein cytokine
erythropoietin, 28
Goodpasture's syndrome,
84–85
granulomatosis with
polyangiitis (GPA), 83

H

hematuria (blood in the urine),
25, 80, 94
hepatorenal syndrome (HRS),
37
HIV and kidney disease,
105–107
HIV-associated immune
complex kidney disease
(HIVICD), 106
HIV-associated nephropathy
(HIVAN), 105
hydralazine, 72
hydrochlorothiazide (HCTZ),
36, 42, 68
hydrocortisone, 92
hydronephrosis, 140

hypertension, 57–72. *See also* blood pressure, natural remedies for; classic blood pressure meds

alpha blockers, 71–72

atypicals, 72

beta blockers, 71

calcium-channel blockers, 70–71

high blood pressure, natural remedies for, 58

hypertensive crisis/urgency/ emergency, 65–68

in pregnancy, 132–133

hypertensive crisis, 66

hypertensive emergency, 3, 67

hypertensive urgency, 3, 66

I

ibuprofen (Advil, Motrin), 33

illegal drugs, 36–38

immunosuppressant medications, 121

immunosuppressive drugs, 81

inferior vena cava (IVC), 8

interstitial nephritis, 33, 37

intracranial aneurysms, 111

intramuscular (IM) application, 21

(intra)renal stage kidney disease, 25

intravenous (IV) application, 21

intravenous (IV) hydration trend, 42–43

isradipine, 67

J

jardiance, 49

K

kidney, 3

alcohol and, 39

anatomy, 8–10

cigarette smoking and, 38

functions, vii–viii

shape of, 8

tobacco and, 38–39

kidney cancers, 113–116

angiomyolipoma, 114–116

renal cell carcinoma, 113–114

kidney disease

basics of, 23–32

polyuria, 25

renal failure, 23–24

stages of, 24–28

(intra)renal, 25

postrenal, 25

prerenal, 25

kidney health, 7–15. *See also* nutrition and kidney health

tips for, 12–15

avoiding tobacco, 13

controlling blood pressure, 13

controlling blood sugar (glucose), 14

exercise, 13

hydration and, 13

sodium and salty foods, 13

kidney stones, 96–98, 137

kidney transplants, 119–127

acute rejection, 122

chronic rejection, 122

References **157**

disadvantages, 119
immunosuppressant
medications, 121
kidney rejection, 122
personal account, 122–127

L
labetalol, 67
lasix (furosemide), 68
levofloxacin, 34
lisinopril (Zestril, Prinivil), 69
loop diuretics, 69
losartan (Cozaar), 69
lupus, 74
lupus nephritis, 80
lymphangioleiomyomatosis, 115

M
magnetic resonance imaging
(MRI), 89
malignant hypertension. *See*
hypertensive crisis
massage effect on blood
pressure, 64–65
metformin, 48
methicillin resistant
Staphylococcus aureus
(MRSA), 35
methotrexate, 84
metoprolol (Lopressor, Toprol),
71
minimal change disease
(MCD), 76–77
minoxidil, 72
monoclonal antibodies, 81
Mounjaro (tirzepatide), 50, 52,
55

Multiple Risk Factor
Intervention Trial, 39
mycophenolate mofetil, 84

N
N-acetylcysteine (NAC), 138
naproxen (Aleve, Naprosyn), 33
nephrolithiasis, 137
nicotine, 38
nifedipine (Procardia), 70
Non-Steroidal Anti-
Inflammatory Drugs
(NSAIDs), 33–34
noradrenaline, 10
norepinephrine, 10
NSAIDs (non-steroidal anti-
inflammatory drugs), 138
nutrition and kidney health,
17–21
vitamin A, 17
vitamin B9 (Folate) and B12,
17–18
vitamin C, 18
vitamin D, 19
deficiency, treatment,
20–21
vitamin D2 and D3, 19
vitamin E, 21

O
olmesartan (Benicar), 69
Ozempic (semaglutide), 50–52, 55

P
parsley tea, 137
penicillins [Amoxicillin,
Augmentin], 78

percutaneous nephrolithotomy, 98
peritoneal dialysis, 29
phendimetrazine, 53
phentermine, 53
pheochromocytomas, 66, 89
plasmapheresis, 85
polycystic kidney disease (PKD), 109–111
  autosomal dominant form (ADPKD), 110
  autosomal recessive form (ARPKD), 110
polyuria (urinary frequency), 25, 94
positron emission tomography (PET) scans, 89
postembolization syndrome, 115
post-infectious glomerulonephritis, 77–78
Postrenal stage kidney disease, 25
post-streptococcal glomerulonephritis (PIGN), 77
prazosin (Minipress), 67, 71
prediabetes, 47–48
prednisolone, 92
preeclampsia/eclampsia, 133
pregnancy and kidneys, 129–135
  dialysis during, 131–132
  gestational hypertension, 132
  hypertension, 132–133
  preeclampsia/eclampsia, 133
  symptoms, 130
prerenal stage kidney disease, 25
propranolol (Inderal), 71
proteinuria, 80
public health emergency definition, vii
pyelonephritis, 33–34, 93, 95
Pyridium, 94

R

ramipril, 69
renal cell carcinoma, 113–114
renal failure, 4, 23–24
renal insufficiency, 4
renin-angiotensin system, 3, 11–12
rhabdomyolysis, 37
rheumatoid arthritis (RA), 82–83
Rogaine©, 72

S

Saxenda, 52, 54
semaglutide, 52, 54
sex hormones, 10
shockwave lithotripsy (SWL), 98
sildenafil, 72
sodium in food and blood pressure, 63–64
sodium-glucose cotransporter-2 (SGLT2) inhibitors, 55–56
Sperati, C. John, 101
spironolactone (Aldactone), 36, 42

References **159**

strep throat, 77
streptococcal pharyngitis
(strep throat), 34
sublingual nifedipine, 67
sugar/the sugars, 4
swelling, 41–43
Swiner, C. Nicole, viii
systemic lupus erythematosus
(SLE), 79–81
ACEIs and ARBs, 81
corticosteroids, 81
dietary changes, 81
diuretics, 81
immunosuppressive drugs,
81
lupus nephritis, 80
monoclonal antibodies, 81

T
tamsulosin (Flomax), 71, 97
tobacco and the kidneys, 38–39
transplants, 119–127
tuberous sclerosis, 115
type 2 diabetes and kidney
disease, 48–50
cure, question of, 49–50

U
unilateral renal agenesis, 138
urinalysis, 25
urinary tract infections, 93–98
kidney stones, 96–98
vesicoureteral reflux (VUR),
95–96
V
valsartan (Diovan), 69
vasculitis, 83

vasodilators, 72
verapamil (Verelan), 70
vesicoureteral reflux (VUR),
95–96
Victoza, 51, 54
vinegar, for high blood
pressure, 59–61
vitamin A, 17
vitamin B9 (folate) and B12,
17–18
vitamin C, 18
vitamin D, 19
deficiency, treatment, 20–21
foods that can increase, 20
vitamin D2 and D3, 19
vitamin E, 21

W
Wegener's granulomatosis, 74,
83–84
Wegovy, 51–52, 54
weight-loss drugs and kidney,
50–55. *See also* GLP-1 drugs
(glucagon-like peptide-1
receptor agonists)
sodium-glucose
cotransporter-2 (SGLT2)
inhibitors, 55–56

Z
Zepbound Tirzepatide, 52

Acknowledgments

Thank you, Lord, for your favor, protection, grace, and mercy.

Sending love to my immediate family, the folks I live with who put up with me: Ric, Price and Blake, thank you for allowing me the space and time to write this book. Thank you to the place where it all began—Swiner Publishing Company. I never would have been noticed by a larger publishing company if it hadn't been for the successful self-publishing ventures I started with at home. I appreciate my mom and dad for encouraging me to focus on reading, writing, and speaking during my childhood, and for participating in the oratorical contests at church that I hated at the time. All of these activities taught me about the importance of my voice, my words, my thoughts, and my ideas. It's crazy how life comes full circle, isn't it?

Thank you to Ulysses Press, my friends and family, and my tribe in real life and online for supporting my efforts and my brand.

Love you forever and ever,

—Nicole

About the Author

Voted in the Top 10 Best Doctors in North Carolina, DocSwiner is a family physician, seven-time best-selling author, speaker, wife, and mother in Durham, North Carolina. She is also affectionately known as "the Superwoman Complex expert" and has written two best-selling books on the topic, which has now evolved into the #nosuperwoman lifestyle brand. She also owns and runs Swiner Publishing Company for authors and entrepreneurs, and Serenity Hydration and Wellness, which provides IV hydration and self-care consults. She is passionate about minority health, women's health, mental health, DEI (diversity, equity, and inclusion), and entrepreneurship.

DocSwiner attended Duke University and went to medical school at the Medical University of South Carolina. She speaks nationally and has appeared on news, media, and as a main stage speaker at Essence Fest and Radio One's Women's Empowerment. She has become one of the nation's experts on self-publishing, media in medicine, self-care, physician burnout, and work-life balance. She has written or freelance edited for online sites, such as WebMD and Byrdie Beauty Brand, and finished a certification at Harvard Medical School through their Media and Medicine graduate program in 2023.

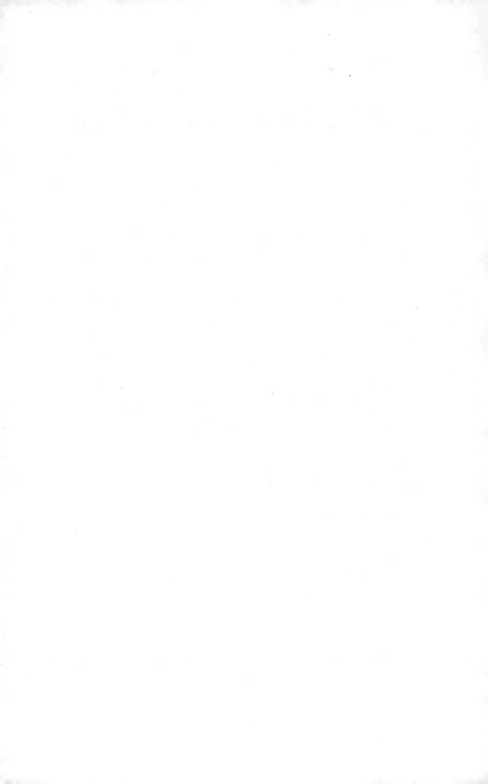